Advance Praise for

Keeping the Home Fires Burning

"*Keeping the Home Fires Burning* is a BLOCKBUSTER all day long. The need is overwhelming for this material. OH MY I'm getting every one of my girlfriends this book."

—Karen Sessoms, Atlanta, GA

"*Keeping the Home Fires Burning* to me...is filled with reasons why I should make love with my partner. I'm learning so much about myself each day. I cannot wait to introduce the new me to him. This book is a great resource guide for me."

—Dawn Love, Lancaster, TX

"Ella gives women additional reasons to accept their sexuality. This book helps women open their minds to great times, and great experiences. It has helped me make important adjustments in my attitude and sensual techniques so that I can be happy in my relationship in and out of the bedroom."

—Bettie Jones, San Diego, CA

"This book is so mentally and physically stimulating. *Keeping the Home Fires Burning* surely awakened my sexuality. It gave me the perfect excuse to be the Diva that I am. This is my passport to be sexy."

—Denella Ri'chard Braxton, Miami, FL

"As I read *Keeping the Home Fires Burning*, I discovered that this is really a great book. It is filled with lots of educational resources and is a great Rite of Passage for women who are between stages of wanting to be grown and need to be grown. It has been my personal guide. I love it."

—Pamela Kennedy, New York, NY

Keeping the Home Fires Burning

A WOMAN'S GUIDE TO GIVING AND RECEIVING PLEASURE

Ella Patterson

A SAVIO REPUBLIC BOOK
An Imprint of Post Hill Press
ISBN: 978-1-64293-477-9
ISBN (eBook): 978-1-64293-478-6

Keeping the Home Fires Burning:
A Woman's Guide to Giving and Receiving Pleasure
© 2020 by Ella Patterson
All Rights Reserved

Cover Design by Cody Corcoran
Illustrations by Larry Strader, Slick Graphics

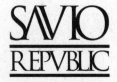

posthillpress.com
New York • Nashville
Published in the United States of America

Dedication

This book is dedicated to the many women and couples who desire to live a lifestyle of love, sensuality, and pleasure.

To the reader—
I hope that you have at least half as much fun in the reading of this book as I have had in the writing.

Sensuous Alert

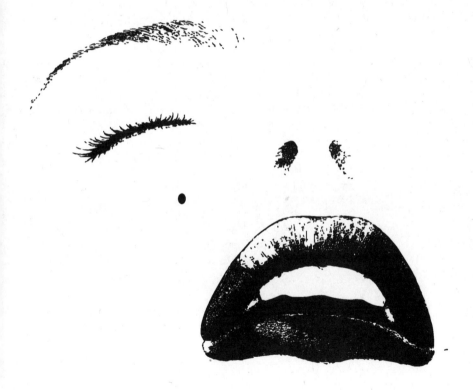

This is a Grown Ass Woman's Book

Contents at a Glance

A Special Note from Ella

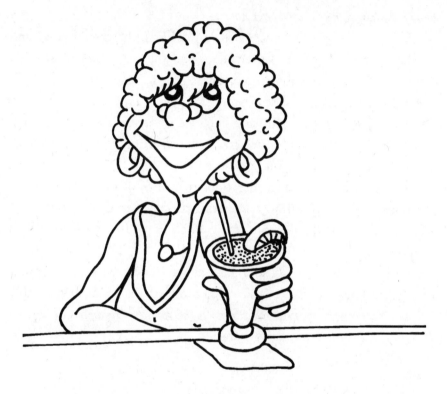

Here women can gain knowledge, incorporate intimacy, enhance romance, embellish beauty, and pursue individual pleasure goals.

Dear reader, this guide offers the sensuous woman numerous ways to enrich her relationships through intimacy and pleasure. It is an easy-to-understand guide for contemporary adult women who want to up their game and become more loving and sensuous as they give and receive pleasure.

The work on this book has been extensive, but it has also been an inspiration for me. Before this book was finished, I found myself interviewing many women, and before our conversations concluded, they were asking me, *"When will this book be available?"* I was embarrassed to say that I did not know because there was still work to be done. *I have been working intensely on a collection of new books—and you're reading one of those books now.*

This book has been one of the most difficult, exhilarating, and fulfilling—as well as one of the wildest and wackiest—adventures that I have experienced. It is organized to resemble a sensuous walk through a woman's sensual life. Use *Keeping the Home Fires Burning* to gain knowledge, incorporate intimacy, enhance romance, embellish beauty, and pursue individual pleasure goals. It will bring great moments of combined joy, happiness, and pleasure.

This healthy and nurturing book presents plenty of fun-loving sensuous tips and techniques for women. Every sexually active adult woman will enjoy the benefits of this book long after she has finished reading.

Join me in a toast. Raise a glass as we honor the positive power of love, intimacy, pleasure, and wholesome sensuality. I now humbly present *Keeping the Home Fires Burning: A Woman's Guide to Giving and Receiving Pleasure.* Now, let's get started.

~Ella

Sex is more than an act of pleasure, it is the ability to be able to feel so close to a person, so connected, so comfortable that it is almost breathtaking to the point you feel you can't take it. And at this moment you're a part of them.

~ Thom Yorke

Preface

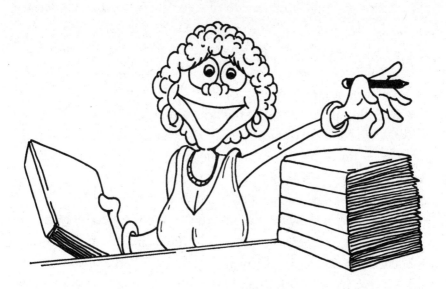

Finally, a Book for Contemporary Sensuous Women

Yes! Finally, a book for sensuous women that is wholesome, educational, sensual, down to earth, and sassy enough to help contemporary women keep their home fires burning. Every growing, maturing, and sensuous woman should have a copy of this book. It endorses the power of love, intimacy, pleasure, and passion. It is for women who believe that healthy sensuality and sexuality are her friends. It encourages positive and uplifting intimate communication for women, rather than an attitude that promotes, despair, devastation, destruction, danger, depression, and disease. This is a fun book that's written in an easy-to-read and easy-to-follow style. It should accommodate all upward-moving sensual women.

Shortly before I began writing this book, something wonderful inside of me began to stir. I was restless and wanted to create pleasing ways in which women could reconcile their authentic sexual selves. It was a challenge at first because, though women want to enhance their sexual aptitude and have enjoyable sex, they do not always admit it.

"I wrote this book with women and their male lovers in mind. But if a woman has a female partner, she should feel free to…try any of the sexual adventures that she desires." It is rare to find a book such as this one—one that provides quality advice about how a woman can incorporate sensual pleasure into her relationship. The techniques in this book are so easy to use that women can make personal adjustments from a drab and uneventful companionship to a sensuous and loving relationship in a matter of hours.

The beauty of *Keeping the Home Fires Burning* is that it makes the secrets of pleasure and sexual loving common knowledge. Written in everyday language, it offers men, women, and couples a manual for navigating the myriads of questions and confusion surrounding intimate relationships.

Included are creative tips and techniques that will help women evolve. Topics include sexual self-esteem, personal appearance, sex talk, sex games, sexual hope chests, sensuality, sexuality, sex toys, sexual lubricants, safe sex habits, and much more. There is also advice and sexual exercises that help a woman's vagina maintain its tightness and gripping power, which in turn can help women achieve heightened pleasure and greater levels of sexual confidence.

Some chapters are purposefully super-short so that the reader can put this book down, practice the sensual techniques, and then go back to where she stopped. Each activity is bulleted or numbered so she can easily find her way back to the place she left off.

WHY WOMEN NEED THIS BOOK

Women who are really smart and conscious human beings sometimes feel like complete idiots when it comes to getting earthshaking, write-home-about-it kind of pleasure. They want their partners to love them in ways that guarantee each loving moment is theirs alone. They want more hands-on passion, commitment, and pleasure from their relationships, but they are not always sure how to get it or give it. They desire the kind of pleasure that is bonding and romantic, and offers a taste of divine peace of mind. They want great feelings that are solid, true, and honest! A woman wants to embark on a fun journey, one that will be beneficial to her as a woman. However, before we begin, here is a summary of each chapter.

HOW TO USE THIS BOOK (CHAPTER SUMMARIES)

This journey is beneficial to women. *Keeping the Home Fires Burning* is easy to understand when broken down into its six major parts. Here is a summary of each part:

Preface, "Finally, an Adult Book for Sensuous Women": The preface of this book endorses the power of love, intimacy, pleasure, and passion. Here, the woman begins to believe that healthy sensuality is her friend. It is definitely for the kind of woman who wants to keep her home fires burning.

Introduction, "Her Portal to Pleasure": The introduction describes how a woman longs for sexual understanding even more than she desires the act of sex. She wants sexual heat to come from a partner who understands her physical, emotional, and sexual needs, and who cares about her along with her pleasures.

Part 1: In Pursuit of Keeping the Home Fires Burning

Chapter 1, "Keeping the Home Fires Burning": In this chapter, we discuss warm to heated moments. Exciting moments that are filled with love, romance, pleasure, communication, and sensuous adventures. Private moments filled with fun, laughter, and excitement. Sensuous moments filled with exploration, rejuvenation, and the attention women long to experience. All of these sensuous moments bring great thoughts and pleasures. Yum.

Chapter 2, "A Sensuous Woman's Body": In this chapter, the reader is a woman on a personal journey. She gets a chance to explore and gain understanding of her own sexual anatomy. To her, sex is more than putting a man's pole into her hole, so she wants to learn how her sex organs work and how to get her body to respond the way she wants it to.

Chapter 3, "His Body": In this chapter, yummy is how she refers to the male body. There is so much to see, touch, and feel when it comes to a man. She loves him and wants to please him enough to make him want to please her. She wants to know more details about his body. The more informed she is, the better her pleasures are. The more she knows about what she can do to make him feel good, the better her sex life will be.

Part 2: How to Improve Her Personal Self

Chapter 4, "Her Feminine Hygiene": In this chapter, she understands that her personal hygiene is important in all her sensuous relationships. Before any woman can wholeheartedly indulge in sensual or sexual activity, she should be very conscious and selective about how and when she cleans her entire body, which includes her vagina, love button, and anus. Each has its own special odor and fragrance, and some have smells that are more alluring than others are.

Chapter 5, "Her Appearance": In this chapter, she will learn that she is a product to be promoted, and she has to make sure she is packaged in the most positive way. It is beneficial to keep her individual appearance up to par. She does not have to be a beauty queen, but she should at least have a pleasing and uplifting personal appearance.

Chapter 6, "Her Sexual Radiance": In this chapter, she will become HER. She has seen *her*, the woman whose face and body would never grace the cover of a fashion magazine, yet all eyes follow her when she enters the room. She notices her because her walk attracts men, exudes confidence, and radiates positive energy. Everything about her says, "I'm hot. I'm desirable, I'm sexy—and I know it." We all know that this kind of self-confidence is great for any woman's ego.

Chapter 7, "Her Mental Foreplay": In this chapter, she learns that her brain is the most erotic part of her body. How and what she thinks will set the tone for wonderful sensuous moments. Her mental foreplay encourages her to feel and act sexy when she is with her lover. Those delicious thoughts of being romantic, touching, feeling, tasting, and of course making sensuous love will light her soul on fire.

Chapter 8, "Her Sensual Conversations": In this chapter, sex is a sensitive conversation that is not always easy for her to talk about, especially when the conversation might include sex games, toys, and intimate interludes. It's important to communicate the positive side of intimate sexuality. Incorporating healthy ideas into her intimate relationship is the goal. This chapter will communicate the importance of sensuous conversations. Nothing is hidden.

Part 3: How to Improve Her Sensuality

Chapter 9, "Her Touch": In this chapter, she will discover that the power of touch cannot be taken for granted. Physical touch is so powerful that it can sway the opinion of the opposite sex and change the previously held judgment and beliefs. All of us—young and old, single or in a relationship—need positive touching. The act of touching communicates more than words. Physical contact is a prerequisite for a healthy individual and for a fulfilling, mature, loving relationship.

Chapter 10, "Her Sexual Rhythm!": In this chapter, she sees how women have tremendous sensual capacity, but many never come close to realizing their true sensual potential. A woman is trained to turn herself off to much of what surrounds her. There are times in her life that she will have to slow down and feel what she is giving and receiving. She can sometimes move too fast and lose her sexual rhythm. She has to maintain her sexual balance. Balance is the key to finding her rhythm.

Chapter 11, "Her Sensuous Kisses": In this chapter, she learns the importance of giving and receiving soul-searching kisses that pique passion, romantic interludes, and the desire to get lost in one another. Kissing is one of the most intimate acts of affection a man and woman can share. To get the home fires burning, start kissing.

Chapter 12, "Celebrating Her Lover's Time": In this chapter, she will come to understand the importance of getting together with her lover for soothing relaxing massages, beauty treatments, great conversation, and good times by hosting a private lover's night-in party. It is easy to turn a normal evening with her lover into a fantastic, intimate celebration.

Chapter 13, "Bring on the Heat": In this chapter, the importance of sharing bedroom moments will become clear to her. A woman's bedroom is her temple of comfort, relaxation, and pleasure. It should include items that embrace sleep or pleasure. It should have a sensuously yummy feel, so that she wants to cuddle, make love, or drift peacefully to sleep. Her bedroom is a place where she renews in the morning and relaxes at the end of each day.

Part 4: Stimulating Pleasures

Chapter 14, "Self-Stimulation for the Woman": In this chapter, she sees that when she needs to get inspired and in the mood, the first and most important thing she wants is for her man to help her get into her sexual zone. Every woman's level of sexuality varies in how she gets ready for love. Whatever it is that makes her feel good and puts her in the mood is what she should do to stimulate her pleasures.

Chapter 15, "Stimulating Her Man": In this chapter, she finds out what every woman should know to stimulate men. She should feel comfortable looking at her man's male identity (penis). I do not mean a short glance; it should *not* be a hurried, surreptitious examination. She should take quality time and talk to him about what he likes. She should plan some kind of treat for him, provided he allows her to do pleasurable things to him. By making it fun, she will enjoy playing erotic games with him and his male identity.

Chapter 16, "Her Gratifying Hand Treats": This chapter will teach her why sex means more than intercourse. It means exploring all the variations that enhance a woman's sex life and keeps it from getting stale. The deeply satisfying power of hand treats is revealed—it is a two-way street, where making her man feel good will make her feel good. Hand treats are fun and give both partners so much pleasure that it is difficult for any woman to fail at recognizing the benefits.

Chapter 17, "Her Gratifying Oral Sex Treats": In this chapter, she will learn more about performing oral sex. She may never like the taste of semen, but over time, she will learn to embrace his naturalness. She will get past all of that and enjoy giving gratifying oral sex.

Chapter 18, "Her Gratifying Quickie Tune-Ups": In this chapter, couples can work as a team to reduce the time it takes to give and receive gratifying sexual tune-ups. Couples can enjoy a sexual quickie when time is limited. They can skip foreplay and move right into sexual intercourse. There are times when a woman just wants to have her sexual way with him and get on with the sex without having to go through the entire foreplay and after play process. It's tune-up time!

Chapter 19, "Her Good Sex": In this chapter, a woman learns how to answer the popular question: when does her sensuality allow her sexuality to take over? It all begins with the woman, but it continues when she is with her lover. Before she looks into his eyes and captures his heart, she has to first catch his eye. Getting good sex is the moral of this story.

Chapter 20, "Her Gratifying Sex Treats": In this chapter, she will realize that to achieve intense sensuous pleasures before, during, and after sex, she should offer delicious treats (sexual treats, of course). Gratifying sex treats help her release inhibitions. She wants to have fun, so adding more to her enjoyment of being a sexually sensuous woman is necessary. Gratifying sex treats are the key.

Chapter 21, "Her Places, Games, and Fantasies": In this chapter, she is asked what more could add to her sexual amusement? Sexy games from sex shops, lingerie stores, catalogs, and the internet. It is about exploring, creating, and sharing intimate places, games, and fantasies that encourage communication, arousal, and pleasure. Adding physical elements of fun to her sex life is key.

Chapter 22, "Her Orgasms": In this chapter, she will discover the truth about orgasms. She will come to understand that there are pleasurable orgasmic experiences for every woman. For a few wonderful seconds she can let go, lose control, and enter a different state of consciousness. It's wonderful and heavenly and mind-blowing—all at the same time.

Part 5: Her Pleasure Containers, Prop Boxes, Hope Chests, and Supplies

Chapter 23, "Her Pleasure Containers": In this chapter, a woman will understand why it is important to have pleasure containers: sexual hope chests, pleasure bags, or goodie drawers. Pleasure containers safely store, hide, and preserve sex toys, lovemaking props, and other sensual supplies. She will see how to make pleasure containers from a variety of decorative cardboard boxes, straw baskets, and plastic or metal containers.

Chapter 24, "Her Sex Toys, Lovers' Props, and Supplies": In this chapter, her sex toys come out of the dark and into the light. Sex toys help her gain a better understanding of her body and heighten her overall sexual experiences with her lover. It is okay and normal to include sex toys, props, and supplies for her private pleasure and sex play. Now go have fun and get it, girl.

Chapter 25, "Her Sensuous Clamps": If a woman thinks sex toys are just for men, this chapter demonstrate that she should think again. They are not! There is a new unbiased world for the sexually interested female, and she has many kinds of sex toys to choose from to heighten all pleasure. There are those that gently constrict and amplify (male identity rings), those that imitate (false vaginas, plastic tits), and those that restrict (bondage implements). For the most part, sex toys buzz or are inserted wherever it feels good. She can get her buzz on too.

Chapter 26, "Her Cyberskin Toys": In this chapter, she learns about toys made of Cyberskin and similar soft, flesh-like materials, which go by various names: Softskin, Ultraskin, Futurotic, and so on. They are made from a high-tech, rubbery polymer or thermal plastic, with silky texture and pliable consistency. They are amazingly lifelike and not cold to the touch, and quickly warm to body temperature.

Chapter 27, "Her Lubricants, Gels, Oils, and Creams": In this chapter, a woman will discover how lubricants, gels, oils, and creams will help her to slip and slide her way to safe sex. There are times when a woman's vagina becomes dry, which makes it difficult to receive easy penetration during lovemaking. It might be time for lubricants, gels, oils, and creams.

Chapter 28, "Her Electricity": In this chapter, we will discuss the emotional intensity that sparks electricity between two lovers. There is also the kind of electricity that is used to excite lovers with safe low-voltage mini-bolts of electricity. The infamous TENS unit machines are small boxes of electro equipment used in physical therapy to send small electrical charges into the skin and relieve physical pain or induce pleasurable sensations.

Part 6: Protect Herself

Chapter 29, "Safe Sex Reminders": In this chapter, knowing that she is protected and does not have a sexually transmitted disease puts her mind at ease. It is sad but true…the days of completely carefree sex have ended. However, there are medical treatments and cures for certain sexually transmitted diseases.

Chapter 30, "Sexually Transmitted Diseases": In this chapter, we will discuss prevention of sexually transmitted diseases (also called STDs, or STIs, sexually transmitted infections). STDs are infections transferred from one person to another through sexual contact. There are over fifteen million cases of sexually transmitted disease reported annually in the United States.

SHARING THIS BOOK

It is best that a woman shares this book with her lover. If a woman suggests that a man read this book, it is important that she provide him loving attention and a sense of care to send him the important message that she wants to improve their sex life. It should not sound too serious to him, and she should not make him feel that he is not good enough or that he needs to do all the work. He will feel insulted and might shut down if she approaches him in this way.

Instead, she should ask him to read this book with her, or she can read it to him. She should tell him how much fun the two of them will have, and mean it. If a woman wishes, they may also take turns reading certain parts to each other.

A man responds eagerly if he feels that the woman really wants to improve her sex life with him. Once he sees the sex improving and how much fun she is having doing it, he will want to participate in the reading and learning process. He will want to help her improve.

If a man does not seem interested, simply leave the book lying around in strategic places that he will visit. His curiosity will motivate him to begin reading. Reading together can help each person become more open when communicating about sensuous things that they would like to try. Another suggestion is that both partners take their own time reading parts of the book they like separately and then come back together to explore what they have read with one another. For passion to grow, it is important that women do not feel they are being judged, criticized, or analyzed for their preferred sexual desires.

HONESTY IS BEST

A woman wants information that is honest, truthful, and straight. If the woman is the type of person who thinks she knows everything, I suspect that this might not be the book for her. She will not be able to absorb the knowledge I am bringing to her. She should put it down or bestow it upon someone more open to enhancing his or her love life. If she is inhibited or feels a little intimidated, then some of the treats, tips, and techniques in this book might not be easy for her to digest. I understand and must be honest with her: this is not a book that seeks to encourage people into believing they should agree with everything I say. It is a book filled with feminine sexual knowledge. It is up to the woman to decide whether she is ready.

My goal is to provide a resource of truthful, honest, and up-front information that can help women make the right choices about what they will and will not need sexually. If a woman prefers, she can take baby steps and soak in a little information at a time, or she can explore a different sensual treat each day. She can enjoy the treats without guilt, shame, or intimidation at her own pace, and she can choose to keep them to herself. She can take a moment and figure out if this is the book she needs and if she decides it is for her, she might want to answer the following questions before reading further.

1. "Do I enjoy making love?"

2. "Am I open enough to try new things with my lover?"

3. "Do I pamper myself on a daily basis?"

4. "Do I know how to pamper myself?"

5. "Am I ready for an intimate and sexual relationship?"

6. "Am I ready to be sexually committed to my partner?"

7. "Do I connect with my partner in ways other than through sex?"

8. "Do I possess positively sensuous attributes?"

9. "Do I practice nonsexual pleasure regularly?"

10. "Do I maintain my sexual ethics?"

11. "Do I bring spirituality into my relationship?"

12. "Does my lover see me as a sensuous person?"

13. "Do I create sensuous moments for my partner and me?"

14. "Are my bedroom activities boring and nonsexual?"

15. "Do I practice feminine hygiene on a daily basis?"

16. "Do I work diligently to enhance my appearance?"

17. "Do I judge people because of their sexual practices?"

18. "Do I combine sensuality with safe sex?"

19. "Do I practice mental foreplay?"

20. "Do I know how to add spark to my conversations?"

These powerful questions need to be considered before any woman begins to understand her sensual self.

A WOMAN HAS TO DO SOMETHING

Every woman must do something to keep her relationship positive, hopeful, and continuously developing. She is responsible for setting up a personal relationship mechanism that will be effective now and in the future. It requires work and confidence-building in order to make the labor worth the efforts. Here are some pleasurable benefits a woman will enjoy:

- ❦ She will take responsibility for and ownership of her personal happiness.
- ❦ She will accept love, give love, share love, and believe that love is her friend.
- ❦ She will learn to express her feelings in understanding ways.
- ❦ She will feel new, alive, whole, and improved by making things better.
- ❦ She will feel sensuously attractive in and out of the bedroom.

WHAT THIS BOOK IS NOT

This book is not judgmental!

There is always something positive she can do to enhance her relationship.

Introduction

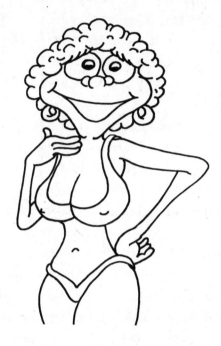

Her Portal to Pleasure

*A woman longs for sexual understanding
even more than she desires the act of sex.*

This book is a woman's gateway to sexual pleasures. It is a portal to pleasure, where a woman can feel free to experience and express her sexuality. A woman longs for sexual understanding even more than she desires sexual intercourse. She wants her sexual heat to come from a partner who understands her physical, emotional, and sexual needs, and who cares deeply about her.

Good sex has positive effects on women. It promotes a sense of care and concern, and can improve her human growth and development. Good sex works wonders for reducing stress and enhancing the human psyche. Positive sexual activity promotes a healthy well-being.

> **Body and Soul**
>
> Answer-seekers often become workaholics, stressaholics, and careaholics judged by society's standards of what it should take to make them happy.

Women who are embarrassed and depressed by their husbands' inability to achieve and maintain erections lose the closeness and pleasure that they once shared. For a woman in this situation, the road ahead is bumpy, and she may not know which way to turn. She needs advice and help. A woman's road to passion is an adventurous one.

When a woman's life is full of stress, she does not always know how to handle the situations she encounters. She becomes desperate and often seeks answers from people who do not know the truth. These answer-seekers often become workaholics, stressaholic's, and careaholic's judged by society's standards of what it should take to make them happy. Searching for the best answers can cause emotions to rise one minute and fall the next, creating an emotional roller coaster. Today the bumpy ride stops. It's time to make the ride smoother.

FINDING HER INTIMATE PLACE

When it is time for a woman to find her intimate place, she can have a friend she trusts take her children to the mall or movies for a few hours. Once the children are taken care of, she can put on her favorite loungewear, prepare her favorite drink, switch off the ringers on her phone, and find a quiet, cozy, and comfortable place where she can read. She can also read to her lover if she chooses. In this private place she has chosen (a place that she can call her intimate space), she will abandon inhibitions and explore her imaginative nature.

A woman can use these handy tips to smoothly transition from one page to the next:

1. Read this book from cover to cover, or dip in and out of different sections for tasty treats whenever the mood strikes.

2. Read this book alone at first, waiting on each surprise to unfold in its own time, naturally and spontaneously.

3. If some of the ideas are exciting but seem too heated, she should not worry—move on, and return to the more tantalizing treats later…when she is ready.

4. If she finds something delicious that she wants to try but is a little nervous about trying it, she can share her desires with her partner and then let nature take its course.

5. Include special treats as she advances her knowledge. There is some space in the back of this book for private notes.

6. Let go of negative feelings, thoughts, or moods that complicate life. Release anxiety by focusing on why a more sensual life is preferred.

7. Take deep breaths often—inhaling then exhaling.

8. Understand that performing sexually is not a priority in becoming a luscious goddess of love, because she is already one.

9. Circle at least fifty sensuous tips and then create a few more to try later. Again, use the spaces in the back of the book to jot them down.

10. Read the directions before using any of the toys, props, or supplies, and check with a professional health expert before attempting any newfound skills this book has to offer.

I hope that these pages through their wisdom and comfort help her discover the sensuous woman she is born to be.

IT IS TIME TO LET GO

These are great times for women to have enjoyable dates, laugh, have fun, and become adventurous. It is time to let go of inhibitions and experience good love. But first, let's answer a few questions that often affect a woman's sexual mood:

1. Is she ashamed of how her body looks? If so, why?

2. Is improving her body image a short- or long-term project?

3. Is it difficult to express her feelings about sex?

4. Is she a sensuous person?

5. Is she romantic?

6. What kind of home would others say she has?

7. Is her home clean, welcome, peaceful, fresh, and pleasant?

8. Does her home denote junkiness or dirtiness? Is it cluttered, smoke filled, odor filled, dusty, or full of unclean allergens?

9. Does her home feel sensuous?

10. Does her bedroom have a cozy, safe feeling?

11. Does she accept how her body feels during sensuous times?

12. Does she know the difference between sex and sexuality?

13. Does she understand her own sensuality?

14. Does she try to make her relationships more sensual than sexual?

15. Does she have good judgment about intimate relationships?

16. Is she comfortable being intimate with her lover?

17. Can she come up with ten creative ways to enhance her sensu-ality? If so, what are they? (These can be listed in the back of this book or in a journal.)

18. Does she find ways to experience more pleasure?

19. Does she give out sensual massages?

20. Does she give herself love at least three times a week?

21. Does she long for the simple or fancy things in life?

22. Is she sensual but hasn't felt sensuous lately?

23. Is she yearning to feel good about her sexuality and power—to be a sensuous woman?

24. Has it been more than 30 days since you she felt truly rested?

25. Has it been more than a week, month, or year since she felt love and concern for a lover?

26. When was the last time the wind blew through her hair?

27. When was the last time she read a good book?

28. When was the last time she received a healing massage?

29. Has she recently walked barefooted outside?

30. Does she want her body, spirit, and attitude to be better?

31. Does her lovemaking need a boost to become what she wants it to be?

32. Does she yearn for a quickie but can't get one?

33. When was the last time she had a romantic dinner?

34. When was the last time she cuddled her lover?

35. Does she yearn for long sex sessions with all the bells and whistles but can't pull it together when the time comes?

36. Does her partner need encouragement to become sexually motivated?

37. Does it feel good to think about sex?

38. Does sex make her feel good during and afterwards?

39. Is she ready to try new things and become more sensuous?

If a woman has answered yes to any of these questions, she definitely needs this book. She will enjoy the pleasures it offers. What follows are loads of solutions, tips, techniques, and treats that will enhance any woman's sex life, improve her understanding, and make her feel better about her own pleasures.

HER PLEASURE IS NECESSARY

Face it, sexual exchange between two loving people creates numerous levels of pleasure. It builds self-esteem, promotes feelings of well-being, and sustains a sense of self-sufficiency. For women, pleasurable sexual exchange provides relief from loneliness, decreases depression, and is a great distraction from pain. It relieves tension, reduces anxiety, and reinforces positive feelings about being a sensuous female. For some women, sex is more than an act of pleasure it's the ability to feel closely connected and comfortable with the person they love. It's so breathtaking that a woman may feel as though she can't handle it at points. In this moment, she feels as if she is a part of a whole. She is in an extraordinary, exclusive experience with an attentive, perceptive, and expressive partner. She is willing to delve into the depths of her soul while sharing absolute bliss in her intimate union. Is that too much for her to ask for?

> ### She Should Know
>
> Pleasure is not about performance or goals. How can she experience the joy of pleasure when she is worrying about her partner or counting orgasms? Pleasure comes when she is relaxed, comfortable with her partner, and with what she is doing with her partner.

That is a pretty tall order to fill for the average man, who gets an erection from a split-second glance at a quasi-sexy image, and then goes through a nearly automated sequence of simple physical motions that culminate in ejaculation. What he wants is the physical passion.

A woman is different—she is more complex. She needs various forms of physical stimulation as well as energetic and emotional connection. She wants her lover to make love to her mind. She wants to feel a sense of recognition, value, and appreciation. If men knew

> ### She Should Know
>
> There is no right way to achieve pleasure. She defines her own pleasure, seeks it out, and then enjoys it to the fullest.

how much better their sex could be with an empowered woman who feels confident, sexy, and passionate, they would certainly be more open to considering what she truly wants in bed.

Guess what: she has to tell him what she wants, and then let him love her if she chooses to receive him. It is up to the woman to lead the way.

ACCEPTING AND RECEIVING PLEASURE

To accept and receive pleasure, a woman has to enhance her ability to receive pleasure. Part of receiving pleasure is being able to accept compliments and affection by letting go of inhibitions and false expectations. By evoking a state of acceptance during lovemaking, sensitivities are enhanced, making a deeper, more profound experience possible for both partners.

Her conscious awareness is her personal discovery of how she will accept pleasure, gradually surrendering to sensitivity with every breath, allowing plenty of time and space to explore with genuine curiosity and a playful attitude. She can guide and direct her partner's attention with subtle body language and responsive sensuality. The more she responds in a positive and engaging way, the more aroused both become, building energy and excitement.

Sex is best when there are no expectations or goals of achievement. Allowing the pleasure of lovemaking to unfold, whether it is the first time together or the five hundredth time, a woman has the ability to set the tone with every movement, expression, and reaction. Achieving optimum pleasure for any woman takes focus.

She Should Know

She is entitled to sexual pleasure. She has not reached her sexual potential because she is not sure what exactly she wants or needs to be sexually satisfied. She must take responsibility for her own pleasure.

Focusing on the physical sensations and feeling present in the moment move the currents of her life force. It surges through her body, revitalizing every cell while balancing her mind and spirit. A woman can practice her lovemaking as a form of meditation—opening her heart to love, enabling her to have more intense, momentous orgasms while sharing bliss with her partner. A healthy sex life can improve other areas of a woman's life as she expands her mind and feels a deeper connection with who she truly is. It feels good when she receives pleasure.

SHE IS THE CEO OF HER PLEASURE

Women want, need, and desire pleasure. She is the CEO of her satisfaction, and she alone defines the kind of pleasure she needs. A woman's pleasure leads to laughter and the rejuvenation of desire and engagement, and it will definitely create a sense of satisfaction even when things in life are going poorly. Pleasure takes the bitchiness out of a woman, even if only for a short while. It softens her, calms her down, and mellows her. She smiles more and is less offensive when pleasure is in her life, especially sexual pleasure.

> **Giving and Receiving**
>
> To have the ultimate sexual experience, she must allow herself to give and receive pleasure.

A woman looks forward to having private, special ways to feel good about who she is. She wants to have the kind of memories that she can recall when she needs to feel good. Great sex is one of the ways of creating those memories.

Women love to be loved, and they like satisfying, mind-blowing sex. They want to define it and seek it without restrictions. There is so much evidence to prove that good sex lengthens life and makes a woman's body feel alive and happy.

Studies have proven that women are less likely to experience a heart attack when they experience good sex with a person they care for. Other studies show that quality sex is great for a woman's health, not to mention it is emotionally satisfying.

While traveling the globe, I have enjoyed speaking to women about the important factors of mutually satisfying sex. I have received thousands of letters and emails from women who wanted more information about the pleasures of sex. Some women confess that even though they have been indulging in sexual activity for decades, they only know the most basic information about sex. Women may be having lots of sex; however, many of them are not feeling the level of pleasure they would ideally like to feel. They want more than bumping and grinding. They

---

Giving and Receiving

Relaxing, receiving, and letting go may be the most difficult parts of sex for some women, but she must do these things if she wants fulfillment.

---

want pleasure that brings magical satisfaction and home-fire-burning kind of sex.

Women harbor an inner sadness when they cannot achieve complete physical satisfaction. This incompleteness makes a woman feel sexually inadequate. Bedroom pressures are overwhelming, and the lack of adequate performance leaves her unfulfilled. This does not mean that sex is the only way to make a woman happy, but many are unhappy and won't be happy until they are sexually satisfied. Women want multiple orgasms. They want orgasms every time they have sex and feel that if they do not have them they have been cheated out of their happy ending. They also feel that they should know every sexual trick that encourages their partners to beg for more.

Pleasure is not about performance or reaching goals. Judging performance sets a woman up to fail long before sex has even begun. Pleasure comes when she is relaxed, confident, and comfortable with her partner's performance. There is not one way to achieve orgasm. There is no wrong or right way either. Even though her partner helps her get there, she ultimately decides what feels good and what makes her desires more sexual. She is the only one who decides whether sex is good for her or good to her.

HER PLEASURE ENHANCEMENTS

Every woman can benefit from pleasure enhancements if she wants to become more in tune with her sexuality. Along the way, she can enjoy some good tips, techniques, and treats to use whenever she is ready.

To significantly enhance her road to pleasure, a woman can:

1. Honor her body. This is important. When she learns to love and honor her body, she is able to enjoy intimate pleasures and fulfilling sensations.

2. Love and appreciate every unique body part. Adore every bump, mole, scar, and imperfection. When she feels good about her physical self, she does not mind coming out from under the covers, turning on the lights, and gazing into her partner's eyes. She understands that there is no perfect body on earth and will begin to accept her good and imperfect parts too.

3. Go on a journey of self-discovery. She takes responsibility for her pleasure and finds out what she likes. She learns to value and discover what turns her on.

4. Share the journey. Once she discovers what turns her on, she shares it with her partner. If she does not know what she wants, she cannot expect her lover to know. She communicates with her partner so that her journey is happier.

5. Relax and receive. While sharing intimate moments with her lover, she can relax her mind and body so that she can also receive love and affection.

She can worry no more…here is her chance to become the sensuous woman she has always wanted to be. Along the way, I offer her an exciting and relaxing journey.

HIS ATTITUDE ABOUT SEX

Many men are unfamiliar with the extent and complexity of their own pleasure. They are not as willing to accept the idea of adding toys to their lovemaking as women are. Dated stigma about toys, stimulation, and personal choices still exists, and men feel like they cannot

> **Heated Moments**
>
> The emotional experience of sex is just as important as the physical experience.

ask questions for fear of appearing uninformed. They know that the penis shaft and head are the most sensitive areas for men, but that information is as outdated as the idea of the clitoris being a little button on top of the vagina.

Men have adopted attitudes and values about sex without thinking whether they truly believe and accept them. It causes confusion and guilt when the woman does not agree with what he morally believes. Exploring both the man's and the woman's sources of information and sexual attitudes can help clarify beliefs. Understanding how the male body works and learning to enjoy it make pleasure better. That is what this book is about…that is the real message: GIVING AND RECEIVING PLEASURE!

SPEND TIME IMPROVING

Women must devote time and effort to self-improvement. Like any other pleasure, self-improvement in every arena helps a woman appreciate her complete sexuality. She needs to love the woman she is and still become the woman she wants to be. She will be promoting herself, and it is up to her to express how great she feels about herself. (Later chapters will show her how to do this without being a braggart.) To become a dynamic "she," a woman must spend time improving, revising, and updating herself on a regular basis.

At times, women are so caught up in taking care of their partners that they neglect taking care of themselves. Oh, they find time to treat themselves to nice dinners, buy new clothes, or go to the beauty shop, but they are not very kind to their inner self. They don't pamper themselves and indulge in the things they enjoy. More often than it feels comfortable to admit, there are women who give so much to others that they become withdrawn from the world and angry at the universe because of what is missing from their own lives. It is time for women to receive the kind of love and pampering that can heal and thrill the soul. It is time for women to take care of number one…themselves.

FOUR PRINCIPLES OF CONNECTING THE DOTS

Before pulling everything together for this book, I had to connect the dots. I needed to find out why women desired heightened sexual pleasure, why some appear to be happy and lead such fulfilling lives, and why others are unhappy and unfulfilled. After long-term observation, I found that women are usually pretty happy, but true happiness came when they were being true to their sensuous self. The happier the woman, the more sensuously satisfied she is.

> **Body and Soul**
>
> Closeness, intimacy, and spiritual connection are the most satisfying aspects of sex. Each person brings unique feelings and experiences to the intimate encounter.

This mission began with speaking to women and asking some of the simplest and the most difficult sexual questions. As I observed and spoke to women, I wrote. The more I wrote, the more I evolved. I gained a better understanding of my own sexuality. As the days passed, I kept writing, and then the better parts of me began to surface. My most sensuous self began to awaken. I realized that like most women, I too was a woman in need of keeping my home fires burning.

> **Heated Moments**
>
> Understanding her feelings as well as those of her partner increases the intimacy and spiritual connection that elevates sex from good to great.

I took stock of what women wanted in order to find their authentic sexual fulfillment. I figured out why some women did not want to have sex with the men they confess to love. I asked, "Was it the woman or the life the woman was living?" Perhaps for the first time, I had to be honest with myself. I needed a simple plan. During this time of introspection, I incorporated four practical, creative, and spiritual principles in my connect-the-dots plan. They are:

1. Establish concrete goals.

2. Get in tune with her sexuality.

3. Make better life choices.

4. Open her mind.

While many of the principles in this book are obvious to some, they are quite absent to others. I suggest that women keep these four simple principles in mind when striving for sexual satisfaction. It is my experience that these principles will add years of happiness, and that alone makes them well worth knowing.

These principles have become the catalyst that helped me write the book that I now present to women. These principles will help a woman define her authentic sexual self and become an important part of her life. Here are four common practices a woman can use to improve her sexual performances.

1. Establish concrete sexuality goals.

Establishing concrete sexuality goals opens up a woman to experience the love in her heart and remember her partner's love. Before moving ahead with any sexual self-improvement venture, a woman has to establish concrete goals.

There are three things a woman does to reach her sexuality goals: First, clearly identify her goals. Second, write down these goals to ensure they exist in a concrete way. Third, affirm them by stating them aloud repeatedly and believing they have already been accomplished. This plan works great for relationship goals too.

Her affirmation might go something like this: "I have learned to do vaginal exercises that will help tighten my vaginal muscles by June 1," or "I have improved my relationship by leaps and bounds and feel very good about my accomplishments," or "I am improving my relationship each week." By expressing her desired outcome in the present tense, she conditions her subconscious mind to accept it as fact. Once she sets her sexuality goals, she can decide what steps she should take to get there. She may decide that learning more about the male and female anatomy provides the best results for her. Maybe improving her personal profile is best, or maybe improving sensuality will get her there the fastest. Could updating her home and its style and mood get her there? Perhaps the section on sexual toys, props, and supplies is her "open sesame." How and when she chooses to become the woman she wants to be is up to her, as long as it brings her the desired results.

> **Body and Soul**
>
> Pleasure takes on many forms: sexual, emotional, physical, happy feelings, sexual satisfaction, bliss, sweet embraces, excitement, new positions, new partner, new experiences, sexual experimenting, or mystery. Pleasure is completely different for each person.

It's important for her to lay out a plan of action. Set goals and then plan carefully for a successful journey. Record the steps involved and then break down the overall process into easily digestible chunks. Practice the ones that work and get rid of those that do not. Take generous bites of those that are satisfying. Creating a detailed plan to improve her sexuality is the best way to reach her sexuality goals.

2. Get in tune with her sexuality.

Getting in tune with her sexuality requires a positive attitude about sex. For a woman to feel attracted to her partner, she needs to feel that he cares as much as she does. A woman will feel defeated in sex if he does not show her that he cares.

Because this is a very sensuous book, I suggest she keep it in her lingerie drawer. She can safely indulge in it at any time she needs a grown woman's book. If any of the treats surprise her—and some of them probably will—she should not become intimidated. She should be a grown-ass woman and open her mind! It's normal to go slowly before trying new sexual treats, and it's okay to feel a little shy at first. She simply needs to read so that she can gain insight and knowledge about how to get in tune with her inner diva.

3. Make the choice to try new things.

When a woman makes the choice to try new things, she must not get bent out of shape or worry about not being ready for this kind of book. Most women who want to learn new things are a little

> **Watch Out**
>
> Sexual pleasure can be a challenge if she is seeking her own sexual nirvana. What works sexually for her friend may not work for her.

hesitant at first, but as time goes by, being comfortable in their skin becomes second nature. Exploring new pleasures becomes a natural part of the learning process. It's the normal order of growing into a sensuous woman. She always has choice before trying new things.

Face the facts: there is no reason to feel guilt or shame for what is sexually enjoyable with her lover. If a woman wants to have fun while being sensuous, she will have to learn how to add the kind of heat that brings elevated spice to her relationship. She does not have to indulge in any of these treats if she does not want to, but she can imagine learning new things that will spice up and strengthen her love life. It makes time together more rewarding and fun.

4. Open her mind.

Women need to free their mind of any negativity and open their minds to the ability to become a knowledgeable, sensual entity. Okay, yes, be an educated, rich, self-sufficient, independent go-getter, but be able to enjoy the idea of having good sex as well. Toss away the mental blocks that are keeping sexual desires null and void. Mental blocks might cause feelings of guilt, fear, shame, pain, or false expectations.

Holding on to resentments or anger with partners current or past is not proactive.

To have the kind of love she desires, she has to work through any negative feelings and bad sexual experiences. Men like it when the woman is happy and able to share in sensuous enthu-

> **Watch Out**
>
> She should not be sexually discouraged. Regardless of her age, sexual history, inhibitions, and other concerns, she can have the sex she desires. She will not find it asking around.

siasm. A man tends to seek the things he needs from another woman if he cannot find it in his partner. Share these tips and techniques, but keep in mind this is not a contest. Use this information to gain wisdom and knowledge. This is the key to living a good life, one that is full of joy and completeness from inside out.

MORE WORDS OF ADVICE

A woman should get a medical checkup before participating in any of the suggested tips, treats, and techniques. She should always do what is best and pass on information that can help others. While exploring *Keeping the Home Fires Burning*, a woman might find that she is being challenged by different personal and sexual habits. She can take her time and move at a rate that feels comfortable.

I wish everyone who reads this book much happiness, excitement, satisfaction, and many *Keeping the Home Fires Burning* moments. This book is a labor of love, and I hope women enjoy reading it as much as I have enjoyed writing it.

Now, to get things really heated, the reader can take this book and go to her special place to get started.

She can always feel more than she can see.

PART 1

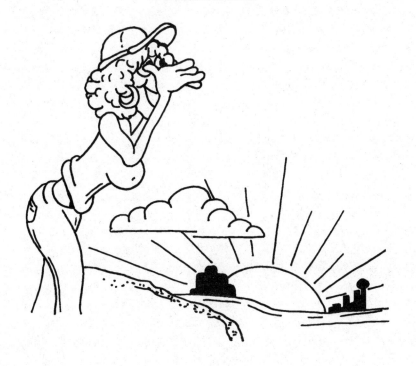

*In Pursuit of Keeping
the Home Fires Burning*

Chapter 1

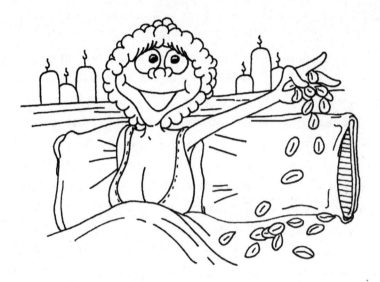

Keeping the
Home Fires Burning

*Sexual pleasure is relaxed and balanced
and nurtures life and well-being.*

Warm and heated moments, exciting moments filled with love, romance, pleasure, communication, and sensuous adventures. Private moments filled with fun, laughter, and excitement. Sensuous moments filled with exploration, rejuvenation, and the kind of attention women long to experience. All these moments feel so good!

The words *keeping the home fires burning* will bring a smile to her face. In my mind, when I hear the word *pleasure*, I immediately think of sensual gratification, sexual indulgences, and great moments of wanted and needed sexual happiness with the person I love.

WHAT ARE "HOME-FIRES-BURNING" MOMENTS?

"Keeping the home fires burning" moments are those moments that include a spectrum of pleasurable feelings from satisfaction to indescribable ecstasy. For some women, it might be that familiar embrace or touch received from a lover. To others it could mean when a lover does sensuous things to her, and he knows what she wants, needs, and desires in order to fulfill her. To some, the fiery pleasure might be the excitement she gets from a new sexual position, new experience, or sensual experiment. To others it might be his passionate tongue flirting from top to bottom on both pairs of her lips, or maybe it is the twinkle in his eye when he is caressing her clitoris with his gentle fingers. Whatever the case may be, these moments are as individual as the woman who is giving or receiving pleasurable gratification. Think: what moments of "keeping the home fires burning" has she experienced?

GET READY FOR NEW PLEASURES

Maybe getting into new pleasures is not her style. Maybe, just maybe, after years of doing things a certain way, she feels that she is finally ready to try new things. Maybe, once upon a time, she didn't think her man would like to indulge in pleasures like getting naked and making love on the patio or in the backyard. Yes, it *sounds* like fun, but she just could not imagine doing it. She could not get past "the nice girls don't do that" thinking.

Now, she is ready. She feels more comfortable about trying new things and is ready to learn more about the things she is interested in. She is ready to share some of these sensuous ideas with her partner and then incorporate some of the intimacies into her love life. She can now kick fear to the side because she is more open to trying a few new things. She is willing to…

- Indulge more in personal and private sensuous games.
- Become intuitive about what makes the body happy.
- Do sensuous things both will enjoy.
- Notice when he is sending hints and ready to try new things too.
- Catch his signs, hints, and messages of what he likes and dislikes.
- Talk about sex in a fun and relaxed tone.
- Always smile when discussing sex.
- Enjoy being sensual by initiating sex.
- Open her mind to new sexual adventures.
- Suggest fun activities that will encourage him to participate.
- Cleary communicate what she wants.
- Listen to his fantasies and enjoy them instead of rejecting them.
- Relay fantasies to him with an open mind.

If she slowly begins to incorporate these treats, she will improve her romantic style. She does not have to be a sexual expert to want more knowledge and information about her own sexuality. She does not have to feel like a nymphomaniac just because she wants to enjoy the type of pleasures that keep her home fires burning. It is time to celebrate her growth.

THIS IS HER CELEBRATION

Even though some women would like to say they do not need to learn more about pleasure, the truth is: we all need to learn more! *She* needs to celebrate *her* pleasurable experiences, especially those that authentically heal *her*. Who a woman really is…is her authentic self,

> **Body and Soul**
>
> She should celebrate her mind, body, and spirit as well as her sexuality. This is her time.

the self that she has always been. It's the core of her emotional and spiritual self. As a woman who is constantly learning about who she is, she should also celebrate her new discoveries!

"Wisdom is a continuous process." It is similar to the human life cycle constantly growing, changing, and forever improving. Rather than marking this celebration with a collection of sexual antidotes, I offer women sensual wisdom that has worked for centuries. "Wisdom is a continuous process."

TIME BRINGS ABOUT A CHANGE

There will be times in a woman's life when sex will not be as fulfilling as she wants. Her desire may deplete, or she may find it difficult to become aroused. Her mind may not be ready when her vagina is, and it may be difficult to imagine achieving a higher level of sexual pleasure. Maybe she's not accustomed to such pleasures. Over time, she may have lost interest in sex.

Sexual pleasures can go downhill because of medications, relationship issues, or life-altering problems that get in the way. Sometimes, how other people judge a woman can affect her sexuality. The good news is this: there is help for almost every problem or dysfunction. We will discuss these options in later chapters of this book.

HOW SENSUOUS WOMEN ARE JUDGED

Some women feel awkward or judged if they cannot find the man of their dreams. Those who are deeply involved with a man and are having sex may feel their minds are sending messages that haunt them during their sexual journey. For example, if a woman in high school enjoyed sex, it meant she was the school slut. In college, she may have been considered the campus whore, and in her grown-up life she might be considered a nymphomaniac. Women are bombarded with so many negative messages about sex and their sexuality that the bad overrides any good she wants to feel. Today we are going to change this way of thinking. Today, she is the only judge that matters. Today she will connect with her emotional investment.

> **She Should Know**
>
> There will be times in her life when sex will not be great. Her mind might say yes, but her body is saying no. The good news is that help is available. This book is a great starting point.

IS SHE EMOTIONALLY CONNECTED?

Many women think sex is better if they are emotionally connected to the person they have sex with. The fact of the matter is…her partner must be just as committed to her emotional needs in order for the fireworks to go off. Sex can be good if there is no emotional connection, but let's face it: in order for sex to be explosive, a woman has to be emotionally invested. Only when she feels safe, honored, and complete is her sexual experience a quality one. There are exciting pleasures ahead for her when she opens her heart to the person she's sharing her love with. She might ask herself if she is emotionally connected and invested in it 100 percent. If she is, she can move on to giving and getting pleasure.

GIVING AND GETTING PLEASURE

Sexual pleasure is a two-way street that must be equally shared. A woman has to be able to give it as well as receive it. This seems simple, but for many women it is a difficult path to follow.

She might find it difficult to open up and accept the wholesome pleasure that she is rightfully due. Some women find it difficult to accept a simple compliment for looking good or for doing something well. Maybe she has witnessed this: like when someone tells her that she looks good or that they like her new dress or new shoes or even that

> **Body and Soul**
>
> Many books are about body parts and positions and its great if she wants fulfilling sexual pleasure, but this book is about much more than that.

her hairstyle looks good, instead of accepting it graciously with a smile, she deflects the compliment and finds fault with herself. If she can't accept simple compliments, she probably finds herself deflecting opportunities to receive pleasure as well.

The training starts today. Accepting gifts when they are offered and compliments when they are given is a natural part of being a woman. She can accept compliments and enjoy them without reservation. The same goes with accepting positive sexual pleasures too.

IT FEELS GOOD TO HER

Today, for many women and men, orgasm has become the epitome of mind-blowing sex. Women are trained to think that if they do not have an orgasm, they are not having satisfying sex. Failure to reach an orgasm may feel like a personal failure for a woman. She blames it on something…her body, herself, her partner, her job, her family, or whatever comes to her mind. She loses so much of herself for the orgasm that if she does not experience it, she resents sex. She then becomes fearful and shuts down certain parts of her sexual spirit.

Let's face it: sometimes she won't be able to see her lover when she wants, and she'll have to accommodate herself. This is where she connects with self-pleasuring. Self-pleasuring is one of the simplest forms of personal gratification. It is as personal and as private as she likes. Women indulge in self-pleasuring through

> **Body and Soul**
>
> Her body is an important part, but NOT the *only* important part of her sexual pleasure. Sexual pleasure is far more complex than the joining of genitals.

masturbation, and many have
decided to use sex toys or fantasizing for pleasure. (see Chapters
14, 18, and 22).

She Should Know

True pleasure is as much an experience of her mind and emotions
as it is her body.

When making love, a woman
should not hold her breath as
she approaches an orgasm. When
she tightens up, an orgasm might happen, but it should happen while
surrendering, losing control so that pleasure can have its way with her.
The more relaxed she is while having an orgasm, the more gratifying
the orgasm will be.

When people are asked how they describe great sex, many will close
their eyes and imagine a satisfying lovemaking session, complete with
foreplay, oral sex, intercourse, and, finally, orgasm. That's what some
say it's all about. Personally, I do not believe an orgasm is an indicator
of great sex. It's very possible to experience intense multiple orgasms
without feeling satisfied. A woman can even experience breathtaking
ecstasy and still not feel satisfied.

To achieve the ultimate pleasure, she should focus on enjoying all
the physical and emotional sensations that are created with her partner.
Imagine fulfillment and then savor how he looks, how his body feels,
how he smells, and how he moves. She should capture the things about
him that she likes when she is holding him. Feel the electricity, relax,
and then release. Have wonderful orgasms. She can come at her own
pace. Orgasms are her choice. Now let it be her who decides when,
where, and how many.

KNOWING WHAT TURNS HER ON

Maybe her turn-on is an indulgent warm bath with water that
envelops her body, letting the ripples of water rubs against her nipples.
It might become a much-needed ritual that she looks forward to
when alone in the bath, or she might consider water flowing from a

removable showerhead that's being used to hit against her clitoris while showering. She might even enjoy walking around in the nude after a long day at work, glancing often at her body as she passes the mirror. It soon becomes pleasurable to relax with who she is. Being able to have cherished moments of sensual freedom is no one's business but hers. She can indulge in private feel-good pleasures without anyone ever knowing. To bring her mind to an area of pleasure, she should ask herself and then answer these questions:

- "What are ways to indulge in sensuous moments?"
- "What are some of my personal fantasies?"
- "Do I consider myself a sensuous woman?"
- "Do others consider me sensuous?"
- "What would it take to bring the sensuous woman inside of me out?"

WHAT SHE WANTS

What a woman really wants is a loving, caring, and attentive partner in her life—one who shows support, love, and affection during her good and bad times. She wants to feel sexy, sensuous, and special all the time, not only when the man is fired up and sexual. Even though she is working diligently to become more sensuous and trying her very best to incorporate more heated moments in her relationships, she sometimes feel that the world is against her.

Men are consumed with getting sexual pleasure from women, so much so that they forget the fact that their relationships require continuous work. They regret being in their relationships, and in turn, they begin to reject their partner's sexual advances. In many cases, the woman feels neglected

---

Giving and Receiving

She should plant firmly in her mind that she deserves pleasure. She should think it and then say it until she believes it.

---

by the person she cares for the most—her partner. Her recurring concern is: "Why is it so difficult to feel good about my sexuality?" Her biggest complaint is: "Men don't try to understand a woman's needs or her sense of sexual prowess." Men equate sex with pleasure, whereas women equate sex with love.

BECOMING A SENSUOUS WOMAN

Does she even know what makes a sensuous woman? Maybe she is not sure of herself. Just in case she is wondering, here are several surefire ways she will know if she is a sensuous woman. Is she…

- The kind of woman who does not mind letting her sexuality shine through?
- Resourceful and powerful about who she is and how she looks?
- Feeling in tune with living a life of happiness?
- In tune with things that appeal to the senses?
- Feeling good about all parts of her life and relationships?
- Confident and comfortable in her own skin?
- A woman who possesses a sensuous quality?
- A woman who knows how to use her gift of sensuality?

Women are committed to finding ways that will enhance their sexuality. It's an important and time-consuming quest. Working to become a sensuous woman is a valuable part of what a woman considers quality time. The best way for any woman to improve her sexuality is to begin first with who she is!

WHY SENSUOUS WOMEN ARE DIFFERENT

Sensuous women are definitely different from other women. They think, act, and treat themselves differently than nonsensuous women. Their differences help them discover new and better ways to express themselves. They find it pleasurable to discuss their sexual desires with their partner. They are always looking for new ways to please themselves.

A sensuous woman pays close attention to a man's subtle clues about what turns him on, and then she sends him easy messages about what she likes. If she is a woman who is having a hard time feeling sensuous, here are some important questions she should ask herself:

1. "Is it simply dinner and back home, feeling distant from my partner?"

2. "Are my evenings spent watching reruns on television?"

3. "Is the only time my lover and I touch when we fall asleep?"

4. "Am I feeling lonely?"

5. "Am I bored with my partner?"

6. "Am I bored with sex?"

7. "Is my love life frustrating and lackluster?"

8. "Am I feeling neglected in my relationship?"

If she answered yes to any of these questions, she might need a sensual adjustment.

CONSTANTLY UPDATE

Women are changing, and it's been a long time coming. They have been changing for the past fifty years while men have looked on. They have changed how they think, work, have fun, and make love. These changes are helping sensuous women make positive strides in their lives, and part of this change has included their sensuality. They update themselves because they want to be better than they already are.

Women are seeking and incorporating techniques that help them become more sensual, but many of them have become goal oriented. They have forgotten how to be successfully sensuous. Don't get me wrong—women are still doing things to become sexier and present themselves as interesting women. They are buying sexier clothes, reading sexier books, and buying sexier products, but that does not make them more sensuous. They are simply sexier...

> **She Should Know**
>
> Pleasure is a woman's right. Her sexual experience will escalate when she firmly believes that pleasure is rightfully hers to enjoy.

and therein lies the problem. A woman has to update her sensuality just as she does her hairstyle and her wardrobe.

Frankly, we all need to work on improving our sensuality. Women work on looking sexy, but they do not work enough on becoming sensuous. Yes, women are sexier, but they have not combined the sexy with the sensuous. Sometimes they don't know how to join the two. They admit their sensuality needs a little updating, and they are working to get more in tune with the new changes they are making. The changes are definitely working in their favor.

WRITING HER OWN SCRIPT

Some women, who have read my books have only been married a few years, some have been married more than twenty years, and then there are those who have never been married. Each group of women enjoyed what they read, and because of this fact, I offer this book as a reminder of things every woman should know.

In it, a woman can find tips, techniques, treats, positions, exercises, games, toys, and all kinds of suggestions and ideas to try. The treats offered are as individual as the women. She should know that not everything is for everyone,

> **She Should Know**
>
> Bad sex is never better than no sex. No woman should settle for bad sex just because she wants to have sex. She is always worthy of good sexual experiences.

and that's okay. A woman should not keep up with how her friends are doing it; she should do her own thing and enjoy what she enjoys.

She should not try to measure her sex life against anyone else's, or use movies, daytime soaps, romance novels, or TV shows as an indicator of what sex should or should not be. She should orchestrate her own sensual interludes and see how delicious sex is.

Don't worry—it only seems kinky the first time she does it.

–Anon

Chapter 2

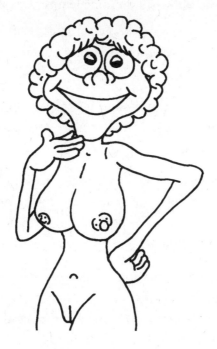

A Sensuous Woman's Body

This chapter will help her love and understand her body.

Because she is a woman on a personal pleasure journey, she should explore her own sexual anatomy. And because sex is more than putting a man's pole into her hole, she needs to understand how her sex organs work and how to get her body to respond the way she wants it to.

To enhance her sexuality, she should understand how her body functions. The best way to learn is to explore her sexual anatomy. This exploratory journey is really a private one just for her alone. She should find a private place where she will not be interrupted and get totally comfortable. It's time for her to do some feminine exploration.

Relax: She gets her favorite beverage. It does not have to an alcoholic beverage. As she starts reading the remaining parts of this book, she should relax.

Breathe: She takes her time and feels her body move into its relaxed state. She breathes, gets comfortable, and then clears the mind for her new education.

Read: She concentrates on what she is reading. She gives herself some time to really indulge and enjoy what she is learning. By not going too fast or rushing through these lessons, she can soak in the information and enjoy the new knowledge.

Think: When ready, she spends time trying each new treat—unafraid and unashamed. This is a book for grown women. She is ready for this, and I know she can take it. She needs it, so she enjoys it in her own time and privacy.

Apply: It is time for her to put the included games, toys, techniques, and lessons to use. She uses them and experiences them as often as she feels the need, as well as thinking of new ways to add the tips, techniques, and toys. This will keep the home fires burning, as she incorporates them with her own grown-folks games.

A woman's body is unlike any other on this planet, so this particular journey will be uniquely pleasant. I will tell her what and where, but she has to look and touch in order to discover her most personal and sensuous self. Remember, this is an exploratory journey. She will have to decide whether to take this journey alone or with her partner. It is up to her. It is always her choice.

WHAT WORKS FOR HER BODY

What works sexually for one woman might not work for another. What feels good to one woman sexually might feel very ridiculous to another woman. One woman might love being naked, but another woman might feel a little shy about the very thought of being unclothed. One woman's idea of passion might be very boring to another woman, yet very exciting to another.

The best way a woman can discover her sexual pleasures is to experiment with her own body, release inhibitions about sexual fulfillment, and then learn what feels good and what does not. She has to open her mind, heart, and body, and remember what she likes and what is best for her!

Every woman deserves a love life that is full, nurturing, wholesome, gratifying, fun, passionate, thrilling, and sensual. It takes a little practice, encouragement, and the desire to get it done. It's that simple. But she must take the journey and get to know herself.

HER PRIVATE PARTS JOURNEY

When we speak of a woman's sexual anatomy, it is referred to as her vagina, but there are many other names women use when describing the vagina. Maybe she has heard of a few of them: punanny, private, snatch, snapping turtle, pussy, poopoo, down there, coochie, crockpot, and cunt, as if its true name is not enough. Part of the reason there are so many names for it is because of the desire to keep it a secret.

As we uncover its identity, we find that the vagina is a very intimate, yet complicated part of a woman, so much so that some women are afraid to play with it or touch it. I think we should explore it in more detail.

The vulva refers to the external sex organs: the clitoris, the labia, the vaginal opening, and the urethra opening. The vagina refers to the internal parts, which include the cervix, the pubic bone, and the urethra.

The Vulva

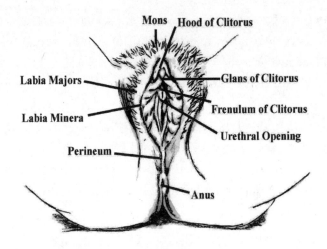

Mons
Hood of Clitorus
Labia Majors
Glans of Clitorus
Labia Minera
Frenulum of Clitorus
Urethral Opening
Perineum
Anus

HER MONS

The first part of her vulva is the mons. The mons is a cushion of fat that sits over the pubic bone and is covered with hair. The skin covering the mons contains many nerves. Touching, licking, and stroking this area can be quite pleasurable. It tends to give her a calming feeling.

HER OUTER LIPS (LABIA MAJORA)

These are the fatty areas on both sides of the vulva that are covered with pubic hair in mature women. They perform a protective role, securing the sensitive structures of the clitoris and vulva that are nestled between the lips. When using vibrating adult toys here, it is exhilarating and provides wonderful feelings of pleasure.

Shaving the labia majora and the mons is common for both hygiene and cosmetic reasons. An extreme form of cosmetic surgery is gaining popularity in which liposuction is used to reduce the labia majora, to open the vulva and leave the inner genitals exposed. One theory is that this ensures the clitoris is exposed to direct stimulation during intercourse, increasing the likelihood of an orgasm. Research suggests this may be true, but I have not tried it, nor found anyone who has.

HER INNER LIPS (LABIA MINORA)

> **Body and Soul**
>
> She deserves to have a love life that's tender, gratifying, sensual, intimate, passionate, thrilling, and fulfilling.

Labia minora are the flaps of delicate flesh that meet the hood of the clitoris at the front of her vulva and run down either side of the vaginal opening. They are nestled between the labia majora, which protect them. Nipping and biting this area becomes so thrilling that it can cause a woman to ooze into a sensuous yet erotic daze.

Size and color of the labia vary enormously from woman to woman. Some women have labia that hang down five or more centimeters from between their labia majora others have labia minora that are tiny and are little more than creases between the inside surface of their labia majora and the vulva. The color is not race related. Her labia can be any shade from light pink to dark brown to deep dark brown, looking almost black, no matter her race. The labia can sometimes darken with age.

Wearing jewelry on the labia minora is increasingly popular, though piercing should be performed by a labia minora expert to reduce risk of infection and damage. Cosmetic surgery on the labia minora is also increasing, though slowly. The most common procedure is the reduction of larger structures or the evening-out of asymmetric pairs of lips. The labia minora is not especially sensitive, though pulling and stretching it can provide a variety of sensations during masturbation. How sensitive is it? The best way for a woman to find out is to experiment without judgment.

The Clitoris

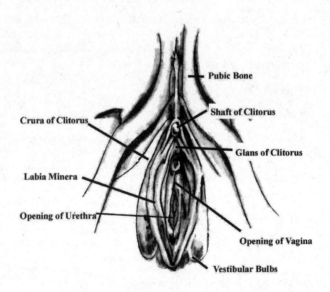

Pubic Bone

Shaft of Clitorus

Crura of Clitorus

Glans of Clitorus

Labia Minera

Opening of Urethra

Opening of Vagina

Vestibular Bulbs

HER CLITORIS

What is it? The clitoris is a small bud-like formation situated where the top of the inner vaginal lips meet. Normally it hides under a small hood of skin, but when sexually aroused it expands and emerges, peeking out like a bright beacon of light in the dark. It is a primary source of erotic stimulation for women. Most women can gain orgasms by gentle massaging of the clitoral area.

HOW BIG IS HER CLITORIS?

It is not very big. While working on this book, I was privileged to see the genitalia of hundreds of women while they were both sexually excited and unexcited. The vast majority of women have an excited clitoris glans (i.e., the visible part of the clitoris at its maximum size is about one-eighth of an inch or three millimeters across, to about three-eighths of an inch or eight millimeters across). Biologically, it's the equivalent to the male penis. Indeed, for the first few months after conception, the genitalia of male and female fetuses appear to be identical. This equivalence is a direct cause of much misunderstanding.

HER URETHRA

The urethra is a tube that connects the urinary tract to the outside of the body. The urethra has an excretory function in both sexes, to pass urine to the outside, and a reproductive function in the male, as a passage for sperm.

HER VAGINA

The vagina is an elastic, muscular tube about four inches (one hundred millimeters) long and one inch (twenty-five millimeters) in diameter that connects the vulva at the outside to the cervical opening of the uterus at the inside. If the woman stands upright, the vaginal tube points in an upward-backward direction and forms an angle of slightly more than forty-five degrees with the uterus. The vaginal opening is at the back (caudal) end of the vulva, behind the opening of the urethra. Above the vagina is the mons veneris. The inside of the vagina is usually pink, as with all internal mucous membranes in mammals.

Length, width, and shape of the vagina may vary. During sexual intercourse or when a woman gives birth, the vagina widens and lengthens up to two to three times its normal size. Vaginal lubrication is provided by glands near the vaginal opening and the cervix, and seeps through the vaginal wall.

FUNCTIONS OF HER VAGINA

The vagina performs the following functions:

- Providing a path for menstrual fluids to leave the body
- Giving birth
- Admitting the male penis for sexual intercourse

HER HYMEN

The hymen is a membrane situated behind the urethral opening—partially covering the vagina in human females, from birth until it is ruptured by sexual intercourse or by any number of other activities, including medical examinations, injury, certain types of exercise, or introduction of a foreign object.

HER PERINEUM

The perineum is the region between the genital area and the anus of both sexes. It is considered one of the most intimate parts of the body. Common nicknames for the perineum area include banus, choad, chode, gooch, gouch, grundel, grundle, and taint.

HER ANUS

The anus is a taboo part of the body and is known by a large number of slang terms, which are generally considered vulgar and not used in polite speech. The human anus is situated between the buttocks, which is posterior to the perineum. It has two anal sphincters: one internal, the other external. These hold the anus closed until time to defecate. One sphincter consists of smooth muscle, and its action is involuntary; the other consists of striated muscle, and its action is voluntary.

Watch Out

Keeping the anus clean is a must at all times.

HER ROLE IN ANAL SEXUALITY

The anus is filled with sensitive nerves that help heighten a woman's erogenous zone. It is said that a woman also feels a small level of pleasure from her bowel movements. It is the release of pressure that gives this kind of satisfactory relief. Anal intercourse can be satisfying to both the giver and the receiver. For women, anal pleasure is stimulation that's shared between the rectum, the vagina, and the G-spot.

For males, the tightness of the anus is a source of pleasure in penetrative anal sex, while the presence of the prostate gland near the rectal wall is a source of pleasure during receptive anal intercourse. Other animals have been observed practicing anal intercourse.

HER EJACULATION AND BODY FLUIDS

Before discussing female ejaculation, let us address the female body fluids in general. Our society views all forms of liquid that is produced by the female body with great disdain. Women are not permitted to openly perform most normal bodily functions; it is not seen as feminine or proper etiquette.

HER BODY FLUIDS AND OUR SOCIETY

Female body fluids are even considered harmful in some societies, where menstruating women are thought to cause crops to fail and livestock to die. This myth creates a problem with sexual pleasure for women in several cultures. Women are expected to maintain a dry, pristine appearance regardless of their current physical activity. Mothers once told their daughters it was unwise to engage in sports, as boys would see them sweaty and disheveled and this would be seen as unattractive. Today, deodorant and antiperspirant ads drive home the idea, "Never let them see you sweat." Women want special or stronger deodorants made just for them. Tampon and sanitary napkin advertising stresses the products' ability to conceal a woman's menstruation from others more than their primary task of absorbing menses or any feminine moistures.

Most women would prefer to have their fingernails ripped out one by one than be seen having a "menstrual accident" in public. There are girls and women who learn to dislike the idea of urinating in a public bathroom and hold their urine all day until they get home. Perhaps they are afraid to be seen as less than pure by others.

HIS AND HER AND BODY FLUIDS

Sweaty men are revered as sexy and virile, and their manhood is measured by their ability to produce large quantities of semen. They write their name in the snow with their urine and see who can piss the farthest. Making a mess with their ejaculate is seen as unavoidable and normal, and these actions are not questioned about men. It is even idolized in adult movies. Men can ejaculate on the face, in the mouth, on the hair, and in the body of their partner, and it is seen as normal. If a woman gets her body fluids on her partner, that is another story—she has made a dirty mess. This is an interesting double standard. If a man can cover his partner with his body fluids, a woman should be able to do the same.

> **She Should Know**
>
> Not all fluids that come from the genitals are semen or menstrual fluid. The obvious example is urine. The body also makes mucus, particularly in response to sexual arousal. This serves an important role in sexual intercourse.

HER VAGINAL LUBRICATION

Female sexuality has been marred by unwritten sexual laws. It is hard to relax and enjoy sex if she is worried about sweating heavily or producing vaginal lubrication. Women who produce large quantities of vaginal lubrication and sweat, and who ejaculate have been known to avoid sex rather than expose their partner or themselves to these fluids.

A woman's desire for sex may increase during her menstrual period, but she may not want to engage in sex during this time because she fears making a mess. Social stigmas concerning female body fluids can significantly restrict female sexuality and pleasure. These fluids are a normal and natural part of a woman's life. There is nothing inherently bad about them. A woman cannot allow herself to ejaculate and experience potentially earth-shattering orgasms if she cannot let go when the pressure or urge to ejaculate arises. As a

> **She Should Know**
>
> Some types of discharge occur in response to infection. Some infections are acquired from sexual contact with a person who is carrying the germ, but many infections are not related to sex at all.

result of the taboos concerning female body fluids, the main motivation behind the studies into female ejaculation appear to be the determination of whether or not the expelled fluid is urine. Do we mean to take this pleasure away from her? If urine squirts at the moment of orgasm, she shouldn't worry. If she ejaculates uncontrollably, so be it. It is not another person's place to judge how her body reacts during sexual pleasure. She gets permission to get wet and messy, have fun, and enjoy sex.

Female Anatomy

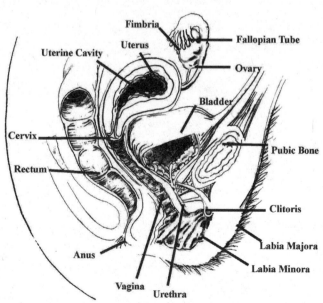

HER CERVIX

The cervix is the slim lower part of the uterus. It connects to the upper part of the vagina. It is a noticeable cone shape that peaks through the upper vaginal wall and can be located with the proper medical tools.

HER UTERUS

The uterus is a hollow, well-built, muscular organ where the fetus develops and is delivered when it is ready to be born. This three-inch pear-shaped area enlarges during pregnancy and is supported by ligaments that extend to the pelvic wall. The uterus resembles a neck that extends downward leading to the vagina. The fallopian tubes are the productive pathways for the ova to reach the uterus. Fertilizations happen in the oviducts, and once the ovum is impregnated, it remains in the uterus, becoming entrenched in the lining of that structure known as the endometrium.

HER FALLOPIAN TUBES

Extending from either side of the uterus to the ovaries are the fallopian tubes. The fallopian tubes carry sperm and eggs that allow fertilization to take place.

HER OVARIES

Ovaries are the ductless glands of the female in which the ova (female reproductive cells) are produced. In vertebrate animals, the ovary also secretes the sex hormones estrogen and progesterone, which control development of the sexual organs and the secondary sexual

She Should Know

Fallopian tubes are an essential part of the menstrual ovulation cycle. Without this part of the female reproductive anatomy, she cannot get pregnant.

characteristics. The interaction between the gonadotropic cells from the pituitary gland and the sex hormones from the ovary controls the monthly cycle of ovulation and menstruation.

Held in place on each side of the uterus are two ovaries, each about the size of an almond. Approximately 500,000 undeveloped eggs exist in the cortex of the ovary at delivery. Beginning at puberty, eggs develop continually, and finally one breaks through the ovarian barrier nearly every 28 days for ovulation to occur, which continues until menopause, or termination of reproductive functioning in the female. After its discharge from the ovary, the ovum is permitted to pass into the oviduct (uterine or fallopian tube) and into the uterus.

HER PELVIC FLOOR MUSCLES

The pelvic floor, or pelvic diaphragm, is a collection of supportive muscle fibers and linked tissue that provides sustenance for a woman's pelvic organs—e.g., the bladder, lower intestines, and the uterus— and it sustains continence as part of the urinary and anal sphincters' endurance.

The urethral sphincter is at least partially responsible for urinary continence in women, but intact vaginal support and levator ani muscular tone also play an important role in female urinary continence. Lost neural support to either the urinary sphincter or levator ani muscle, or lost vaginal support, can contribute to an individual woman's urinary incontinence problems.

Some of the problems that contribute to pelvic organ prolapse are age, childbirth, family history, and hormones. The most shared opinion that prolapse is influenced by the absence of "fascial" support is tough to support with the available current evidence. The vagina dangles by connectors to the perineum, pelvic sidewall, and sacrum via attachments that have collagen, elastin, and smooth muscle. Repair of absent or lacking vaginal support may involve surgery.

HER SKIN

Skin is a pathway to sensuous pleasure. Every body part with skin has a chance of being a pleasure zone. Her nerves respond to touching, stroking, massaging, sucking, and kissing.

HER BREASTS

The breasts are covered by skin; each breast has one nipple surrounded by the areola. The areola is colored from pink to dark brown, is hairless, and has several sebaceous glands. The larger mammary glands within the breast produce milk; they consist of several lobules, and each breast has some ten to twenty lactiferous ducts that drain milk from the lobules to the nipple, where each duct has an opening.

She is imperfect, permanently and inevitably flawed.
And she is beautiful.

–Amy Bloom

Chapter 3

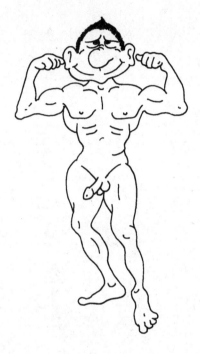

His Body

"You have to be able to center yourself, to let all of your emotions go. Don't ever forget that you play with your soul as well as your body."

- Kareem Abdul-Jabbar

Yummy is how women refer to the male body. There is so much to see, touch, and feel when it comes to a man. If she loves her lover and she wants to please him enough to make him want to please her more, she should know some details about his body. The more informed she is, the better her pleasures will be. The more she knows about what she can do to make him feel good, the better her sex life will be.

HIS PENIS

The human penis is made up of three columns of erectile tissue that is arranged crossways. A free fold of skin protects the corpus spongiosum. There are two corpora cavernosa and one corpus spongiosum that form the extremity.

The Perineum

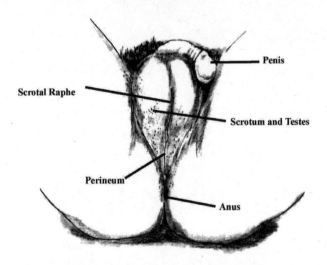

The corpus spongiosum lies on the underside (known also as the ventral side) of the penis; the two corpora cavernosa lie next to each other on the upper dorsal side. The end of the corpus spongiosum is enlarged and cone shaped, and forms the glans penis. The glans supports the foreskin, or prepuce, a loose fold of skin that in adults can retract to expose the glans. The area on the underside of the penis, where the foreskin is attached is called the frenum or frenulum.

The urethra is the final part of the urinary tract and crisscrosses the corpus spongiosum. The opening hole at the tip of the penis is the meatus, and it is where the urine and ejaculation of semen are released. Sperm is produced in the testes, stored in the epididymis, and released through the meatus of the penis.

During ejaculation, sperm propels up the vas deferens, two ducts that pass over and behind the bladder. Fluids are added by the seminal vesicles, and the vas deferens turns into the ejaculatory ducts, which join the urethra inside the prostate gland. The prostate and the urethral bulb add further secretions. Semen is released through the penis.

Raphe is the ridge that looks like a long vein running between the lateral halves of the penis and is located underneath the penis. It runs from the opening of the urethra to the perineum, the area between the scrotum and anus.

The Penis

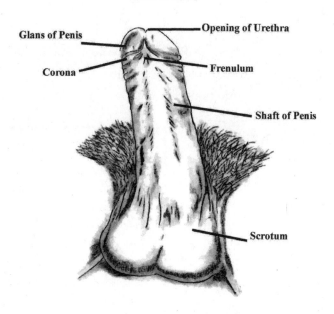

75

HIS ERECTION

Erection is the stiffening and rising of the penis, which occurs in the sexually aroused male, though it can happen in nonsexual situations. The primary physiological mechanism that brings about erection is the autonomic dilation of arteries supplying blood to the penis, which allows more blood to fill the three spongy erectile tissue chambers in the penis, causing it to lengthen and stiffen. The now-engorged erectile tissue presses against and constricts the veins that carry blood away from the penis. More blood enters the penis than leaves until equilibrium is reached (equal volume of blood flowing into the dilated arteries and out of the constricted veins). A constant erectile size is achieved at equilibrium. Erection facilitates sexual intercourse, though it is not essential for some other sexual activities. Although many erect penises point upwards (see illustration), it is common and normal for the erect penis to point nearly vertically upwards or nearly vertically downwards, depending on the tension of the suspensory ligament that holds it in position. Stiffness of erectile angle also varies.

HIS PERINEUM

The perineum corresponds to the outlet of the pelvis. Its deep boundaries are—in front, the pubic arch and the arcuate ligament of the pubis; behind, the tip of the coccyx; and on either side, the inferior rami of the pubis and ischium, and the sacrotuberous ligament.

The perineum is the area between the base of the penis and the anus. The bulb of the penis is in this area, but deeper inside the body. The prostate gland is found even

---

She Should Know

When kissing and caressing, she should not forget to also stimulate the perineum and delicately massage this area with the tip of the finger. Then, she should watch his reaction. She shouldn't do it for too long. She should alternate with other movements, and then come back to devote special attention to this spot.

---

deeper. The perineum is identified by the line drawn straight down the middle. It is highly sensitive when it is stroked or massaged.

The space is tablet shaped and partially on the surface of the male's scrotum or the female's vulva. It is located by the buttock's rear and by the medial side of the thigh. There is a line crossway across the ischial tuberosities that divides the space in halves. Located at the posterior end of the anal canal is the anal region. The anterior region embodies the external urogenital organs region. When a woman gently strokes or massages this area, it creates pleasurable sensations for her partner.

Male Reproductive System

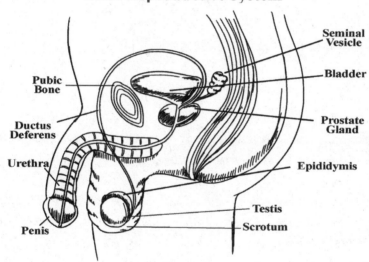

HIS TESTES/TESTICLES

The male gonads, also called testes or testicles, grow in the abdominal cavity. Two months before birth, or shortly after birth, the testes drop through the inguinal canal into the scrotum and then into a sack that spreads below the abdomen, behind the penis. This location makes them susceptible to injury.

Each testis is an egg-shaped structure about five centimeters long and three centimeters in diameter. A hard, white, rubbery, connective tissue capsule, the tunica albuginea, surrounds each testis and is drawn inward to form septa that divide the organ into lobules. There are approximately 250 lobules in each testis containing one to four coiled sperm producing tubules that unite to form one straight tubule, leading into the rete testis. Short efferent ducts leave the testes. Interstitial cells promote the production of male sex hormones and are located in the body fluids.

> **Body and Soul**
>
> Testicles hang outside the body because the ideal temperature for sperm production should be one to two degrees lower than body temperature. In situations where men get cold, testicles get closer to the body.

HIS SCROTUM

The scrotum is an external bag of skin and muscle containing the testicles. It is an extension of the abdomen and is located between the penis and the anus. The female homologue during fetal development is the labia majora.

The scrotum keeps the testicles' temperature about 3 degrees Celsius lower than that of the rest of the body. The best testicle temperature is around 34.4 degrees Celsius (94 degrees Fahrenheit). When a man's temperature is too much above or too much below 94 degrees Fahrenheit, it may be damaging to his sperm count. The temperature is regulated by moving the testicles closer to the abdomen when it is cold and away when hot. When sexually aroused or too cold, the muscle contracts and pulls the testes closer to the body for warmth. The scrotum consists of skin and subcutaneous tissue. A vertical divider of tissue in the center separates it into two parts, each containing one testis. Muscle tissue contracts to give the scrotum its wrinkled appearance, but when relaxed, the scrotum is smooth. The cremaster muscle has skeletal muscle fibers that control the position of the scrotum and testes.

HIS PROSTATE

The prostate is an exocrine gland of the male mammalian reproductive system. Its main function is to secrete and store a clear, slightly basic fluid that constitutes up to one-third of the volume of semen. The prostate differs considerably between species anatomically, chemically, and physiologically. A healthy human prostate is slightly larger than a walnut. It surrounds the urethra just below the urinary tract. It is located in front of the rectum and is felt during a rectal exam.

HIS URETHRA

The male urethra has two functions: to carry urine from the bladder during urination and to carry semen during ejaculation. Within the prostate, the urethra coming from the bladder is the prostatic urethra and merges with the two ejaculatory ducts. Semen comprises sperm and seminal fluid; some of the seminal fluid is produced by the prostate gland, and the rest is produced by the two seminal vesicles. The prostate also contains some smooth muscle that helps to expel semen during ejaculation.

Prostatic secretions are generally made up of simple sugars and are often slightly basic. In human prostatic secretions, the protein content is less than 1 percent and includes proteolytic enzymes, acid phosphatase, and prostate-specific antigens. Its secretions contain zinc and citric acid.

To work properly, the prostate needs male hormones (androgens). Male hormones are responsible for male sex characteristics. The main male hormone is testosterone, which is produced mainly by the testicles. Some male hormones are produced in small amounts by the adrenal glands. Prostate glands are only in males; Skene's glands in females are homologous to the prostate gland in males.

HIS BREASTS

The male breasts are essentially nipples with surrounding areola. A man does not have the fat and glands that a woman has—the tissue that gives a woman her cup size—but like ours, his nipples are very sensitive and become more sensitive when he becomes aroused. A few men can experience orgasm when aroused by their breasts.

WHAT HAPPENS DURING HIS ERECTION

Erection happens during arousal—one of the phases of the sexual response cycle. A number of changes in the body happen during this phase. In both men and women, the heart begins to beat faster and blood pressure rises. The muscles in the body grow tense, and the nipples may get hard. People may have what is called a "sex flush" — they redden around the chest and neck.

Increased blood flowing to the genitals will cause the penis to become erect, and guys will notice their testicles drawing closer to their body as the scrotum thickens. In girls, breasts enlarge, the vagina lubricates, and the clitoris begins to swell.

Body and Soul

Men generally have their penis straight hanging to either side. This is because the testicles are unequal, meaning one is higher than the other. When the penis is erect, it's not a straight line and is more noticeable than usual, but she doesn't have to worry. It's a normal thing found in most men.

The penis and the clitoris are very similar. They are both made of spongy erectile tissue and are full of sensitive nerve endings. The penis extends out from the body for several inches. The clitoris extends into the body for several inches. Like men, women get erections, but they're not as noticeable.

HIS EJACULATION AND ORGASM

Ejaculation is the process of ejecting semen from the penis and is usually accompanied by orgasm as a result of sexual stimulation. It may also occur spontaneously during sleep (called a nocturnal emission), due to stimulating of the prostate or, rarely, due to prostatic disease.

His ejaculation is a reflex that cannot be stopped without painful cramping once it has started. It has two phases: emission and ejaculation proper. During emission, the two ducts known as vas deferens contract to propel sperm from the epididymis (where it was stored) up to the ampullae at the top end of the vas deferens. The beginning of emission is experienced as a "point of no return." The sperm then passes through the ejaculatory ducts and is mixed with fluids from the seminal vesicle, the

---

Body and Soul

Good news! She can determine when her lover has an orgasm just by looking at his testicles. They rise slightly just before ejaculation to "connect" with his body, and she can take advantage of this chance, enhancing its pleasure by methods known only by her.

---

prostate, and the bulb urethral glands to form the semen, or ejaculate. During ejaculation proper, the semen is ejected through the urethra with rhythmical contractions.

The energy and quantity of ejaculate differ for each male. One man may produce anywhere from two to fifteen milliliters while another man may produce two to six milliliters of ejaculate. Ejaculate measurements are affected by the amount of time that has passed since his last ejaculation. Larger ejaculate measurements are helpful with abstinence. The length of the stimulation leading up to the ejaculation can affect the volume. When a man experiences abnormally low volume, it is hypospermia.

The number of sperm in an ejaculation varies due to the timing of last ejaculation, temperature of testicles, level of sexual excitement prior to ejaculation, age, testosterone level, general fertility, and volume of seminal fluid. An unusually low sperm count is not the same as low semen volume. Low semen volume is known as azoospermia.

The ejaculation reflex is caused by the sympathetic nervous system, while erection of the penis is caused by the parasympathetic nervous system. Most men experience a lag time of a half hour or so between the ability to ejaculate consecutively. During this refractory period, it is difficult or impossible to attain an erection, because the sympathetic nervous system counteracts the effects of the parasympathetic nervous system.

There are wide variations in how long sexual intercourse can last before ejaculation occurs. Studies have shown that most men can only

---

Body and Soul

Are blue balls a myth? Blue testicles occur when a man is excited for a long time without orgasm. The blood accumulated in the testicles remains there, and because it doesn't have oxygen, the testicles swell and become blue.

---

avoid ejaculation during active thrusting for five minutes or less. A minority can ejaculate more or less at will and delay ejaculation for an hour or longer during sexual intercourse.

At the conclusion of sexual intercourse, most men ejaculate while inside their partner. However, some prefer to withdraw their penis from their partner's body and ejaculate elsewhere, such as on their partner's face or chest. This is coitus interruptus. Ejaculation can also occur during oral sex, where the man's partner orally stimulates his penis. Ejaculation can occur in the partner's mouth, or he can withdraw from the mouth and ejaculate on the face or other parts of the body. This type of ejaculation is just as enjoyable as ejaculating inside the mouth, vagina, or anus.

When a man ejaculates before he wants to it is called premature ejaculation. If a man is unable to ejaculate in a timely manner after prolonged sexual stimulation, in spite of his desire to do so, it is called impotence.

Never cease to explore new ways and methods of improving.

PART 2

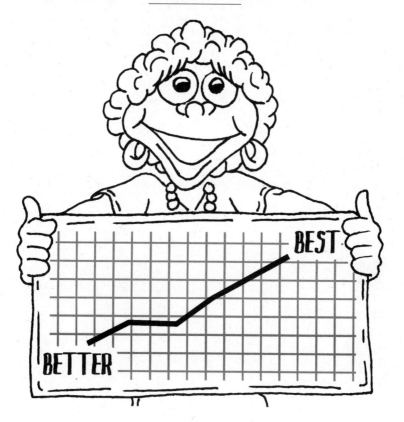

How to Improve Her
Personal Self

Chapter 4

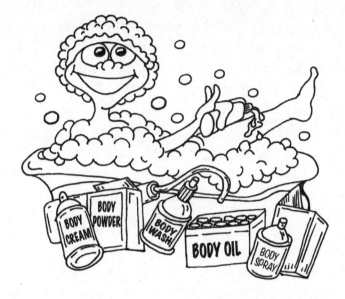

Her Feminine Hygiene

Every woman's body odor is unique. No two are the same.
Just as fingerprints, they are different.

A woman should become committed to excellent feminine hygiene. No matter what age she is or what she likes to do with her genitals, keeping herself healthy is top priority. There are many simple ways to keep the most essential part of her anatomy healthy. Incorporating feminine hygiene into her daily routine will keep it happy, allowing her to enjoy a more comfortable and healthier life.

1. Choose intimate materials that are kind.

   Shopping for panties is usually an exciting activity, but the vagina will start crying if it cannot breathe. Avoiding nylon and wearing cotton are best. Cotton allows her private parts to breathe, whereas nylon inspires them to sweat and retains fluids against the skin. Water retention is fantastic when going for a swim, but it's safe to assume she's not underwater most of the time. Nylon could lead to candidiasis—aka thrush. In contrast, cotton allows the vagina to breathe, reduces sweat, and therefore provides less room for bacteria to form and proliferate. Not only does the vagina feel comfortable, but also the vulva breathes a sigh of relief.

2. Update the wiping technique.

   Women have been wiping after going to the toilet for years, so it's fair to assume women are pros, right? Alternatively, maybe not...Cystitis often crops up because of bacteria that live in the colon making its way to the urethra—the hole women pee through. Since it does not belong there, it can cause urinary tract infections (UTIs). One of the easiest ways to avoid UTIs is to wipe from top to bottom (front to back), not bottom to top (back to front). If a woman is already doing this, that means she is experienced at it. If not, now's the time to make the change and follow this new technique!

3. Avoid soap for pH balance.

   Toxic shock syndrome (TSS) is a serious bacterial infection that can set in a little easier if the vagina's pH isn't steady or in balance. The vagina is a delicate area, and it is not to be messed with. Avoiding soap is the best way to keep these kinds of infections away. Certain soaps disrupt the vaginal pH and wash away the "friendly" bacteria called lactobacilli. As lactobacilli exist in part to combat any bad invaders, such as staph aureus, a woman needs to keep them happy. So what's best to use? Water. Water is the best medicine for her vagina area. Its neutral pH lends itself well to keeping lactobacilli happy, which in turn keeps her vagina healthy.

4. Douching is not necessary.

    Back in the Victorian era, douching was all the rage. In fact, Queen Victoria herself used it as a means of engaging in feminine hygiene. Since then, science has proven that douching is harmful. A recent analysis of the douching practice shows that vaginal douching increases a woman's risk of developing bacterial vaginosis by one to five times. On the scarier side of things, douching increases the risk of cervical cancer. A popular reason for using vaginal douching is to clear away menstrual blood, in an attempt to stay fresh during her period. A better way for her to approach this is to run clean water over the vulva/external genitalia, change tampons regularly, and wear breathable panties. Lukewarm water is best if she must douche.

5. Take a safe approach to shaving down below.

    Shaving is all the rage these days, and rage is what her privates will feel if a woman does not do it right. According to girlshealth.gov, pubic hair plays an important role in protecting the labia against scratches, nicks, cuts, and abrasions. She may want to consider trimming rather than a full shave. On the other hand, shaving often heightens sensations for women. If she decides to shave it all away, she can try the following:

Ella Patterson

Do it in the shower but toward the end of the shower when her pores are open. This makes it easier for hairs to be removed. She should always use a brand-new, clean razor and never share razors. Sharing increases the risk of catching a blood-borne virus from someone else. Use of a shaving cream or lubricating gel will reduce the friction between the razor and the vulva. This reduces the risk of cuts. She should go slowly and not rush the process. Avoiding a cut is key. Cuts act as a point of entry for bacteria. The vulva is not a fun place to have a cut-related infection. Please take care.

6. Get to know the healthy vaginal scent.

   This may sound a little crazy at first, but getting to know the vaginal scent and sensations allows a woman to learn when something is wrong. When does a woman know something is wrong? If she starts to smell different, secrete a discharge that is not clear or white, or simply feel a little uncomfortable, she should visit her gynecologist or primary care provider. Symptoms such as abnormal vaginal discharge and strong odor could be signs of various infections.

7. Use a lubricant.

   Vaginal dryness can occur for a whole host of reasons. It is predominantly caused by a decrease in estrogen. While menopause commonly leads estrogen levels to drop, in some cases, stress, depression, chemotherapy, and intense exercise, among other things, could play a role. If this happens, a woman's sexual drive or desire to have sex might fall. If she is simply not up for it, that is fine. However, if it's vaginal dryness holding her back, there is an answer. Using a lubricant allows her

88

to enjoy sex without discomfort. Using one that's pH friendly (see Chapter 27, "Her Lubricants, Gels, Oils, and Creams") keeps her vaginal canal happy. Doing this reduces the risk of internal cuts, allowing her to enjoy sex safely.

8. Practice safe sex.

    Unless she is in a relationship where both parties have been given the all-clear by a sexual health specialist (or other medical specialist), a woman should use barrier contraceptive. (see Chapter 29, "Safe Sex Reminders"). The same applies to any oral activities, because such diseases as gonorrhea or herpes can also spread that way. The American Sexual Health Association estimates that one in two adults will contract an STI by their mid-twenties. Engaging in safe sex prevents a woman from becoming part of that statistic. For any other question, please speak to a medical professional. This advice is written solely for informative purposes and should not be a replacement for a medical specialist's advice.

UNDERSTANDING HER HYGIENE

Okay, okay…I know I mentioned basic hygiene in my last book, but I received so many letters and emails about how great the information was that I thought I should expand on the subject in this book. Come on—women need it. Mature women understand that hygiene is important in all sensuous relationships. Before any woman can wholeheartedly indulge in sensual or sexual activity, she should consider the importance of her personal hygiene.

COMMON CAUSES OF HER BODY ODORS

Every woman's body odor is unique. No two smell the same. Just as fingerprints are different, so is everyone's body odor. There are common factors associated with body odors, so a woman should get in tune with her body to find out if and why she has any bothersome odors. She should be very conscious and selective about how and when she cleans her entire body, which includes her vagina, love button, and anus. Each has its own special odor and fragrance, and some will have smells that are more alluring than others are:

Some common reasons for feminine odors are:

- Diet and eating habits
- Medications
- Exercise programs
- Rest factors
- Body oils/perfumes
- Lotions and powders
- Water source
- Soap products
- Skin type
- Body condition
- Body functions
- Masturbation habits
- Masturbation fluids
- Vagina secretions
- Menstrual cycle
- Urine residue
- Frequency of sex
- Physical activity
- Female maintenance

CLEANING HER VAGINA

Douching is not always necessary to keep her vagina clean. The normal, healthy vagina naturally cleans itself, but a woman must help it. If she feels it is necessary to douche after her period, she can do so with little worry of developing problems. Women who douche too frequently can destroy the colonies of beneficial bacteria that normally inhabit the vagina, leaving it vulnerable to organisms that cause vaginitis (inflammation of the vagina).

Some women douche too much because they smell unpleasant odors or experience excessive discharges. The normal vagina will not have a continuous bad odor or excessive discharge. An odor exists when an infection is present. Unhealthy odors in the vaginal region equal an unhealthy vagina.

> **She Should Know**
>
> Women don't need to douche. The vagina is a self-cleaning organ. When she tries to clean it by using douche, she actually flushes away normal, healthy microbes as well as temporarily changing the pH nature of the vagina.

Good personal hygiene makes the woman more attractive and her sex more alluring. She does not need to douche in preparation for sex if she has washed her external vagina area carefully. Using gentle soapy hands to wash the outside of the vagina is a favorite of most women. A woman can apply a dash of perfume or fragrance on the inner thighs or slightly above her panty line to add sensual allure. She will appreciate it, and her lover will love it. Perfumes that are light and pleasant, not too spicy or strong, are best. A woman does not want her lover to enjoy her smell and hate her taste because she has over sprayed.

CLEANSING HER CLITORIS (LOVE BUTTON)

The clitoris is rarely mentioned when speaking about cleaning the sex organs, but it needs proper cleaning too. Located at the head of the vagina and covered by fluffy skin under the labia, the clitoris stands

She Should Do

If she wants to look beautiful, it's not enough to just put on some makeup and dress according to the latest fashion trends. She must take care of her body and personal hygiene. Not only will that give her an aura of freshness, but it will also help her stay healthy and battle infections.

to be dealt with in more ways than one.

The clitoris is called the love button due to its sensitive nature in helping women achieve orgasms. To clean it, a woman should pull the skin of the labia back and then, using circular motions with a swab, gently remove any mucus buildup that is embedded there. She should not over clean it, because the natural secretions of this orifice are sensuous and healthy—they help the clitoris work smoothly. But she does not want the mucus to build up.

A woman would only want to cleanse the clitoris after lovemaking or after her monthly period has ended. Sometimes the fluids from sex and menstrual detritus will hide inside the skin folds of her love button, causing nasty odors that are rarely detected and never cleaned. Bacteria and unwanted odors are difficult to detect because women never look for them there. Her partner will be able to smell any signs of foul odor as soon as he gets near her. The main thing to remember is she must keep her body and clitoris clean and fresh.

CLEANSING HER ANUS

The anus should be cleaned just as any other part of her body. Wiping once with tissue after a bowel movement isn't enough to say that it is thoroughly cleaned. More time and care should be given to cleaning it correctly. One way to clean the anus better is to wipe properly from front to back several times after a bowel movement.

Women have personal accessories included in their douche packets that are provided to clean the anus, but men are left to dig, pull, and wipe endlessly, only to share their skid marks with the rest of the wash.

A woman should cup the tissue and wipe again, even if she thinks she has cleaned all residue. Wiping twice for practical reasons may cause a woman to use more tissue than normal, but it is worth it to feel clean. She can use fragrance-free baby wipes if needed.

I have gone to great lengths to find the answer to an obvious but well-kept secret: "Why do men have bowel streaks in their underwear on a regular basis?" My theory is the number of times men actually sit down to use the commode is fewer than women do. Therefore, women wipe their anus more often than men do. The fact is, men stand while urinating while women sit; therefore, women wipe twice as much as men. Women are also taught and trained to wipe from the front to back after each toilet use, which leads me to believe that we actually wipe our anus with almost every toilet use. Each woman I interviewed said that almost every time she used the toilet, she wiped her anus, whether intentionally or not. It was primarily a habitual reflex. Physical evidence proves that men are susceptible to producing long-time streaks in their underwear far more than women.

HYGIENE AND BATHING

During a woman's me-time moments, she can pamper her feminine area more than she would with her regular regimen. When preparing for a hot sexual encounter, nothing works like pre-sex hygiene. Prior to sex, she can sit in a very warm bath or, if available, soak in a Jacuzzi. The increased stimulation from the jets will enhance the effects of the warm water as it helps clean her skin and private parts. If she does not have time for a bath, she can take a warm, moist washcloth and wipe gently over her vulva for a few minutes. After a long session of good sex, she can fill a hot water bottle with warm water and sit on it or lie down and rest her vulva and love button on it.

Maybe she wants to share a bath with him. Alternatively, she can wrap a clean, thick, warm, moist hand towel around his penis before a hand- or blowjob. It will relax and freshen him while getting him ready for lovemaking. It's great, and he'll love it!

BATHING TO STIMULATE

Any bath can be sensually stimulating and lead to other fulfilling moments. A woman's mind, body, and love life will benefit from these stimulating baths. These kinds of baths are great for promoting basic hygiene.

She will need steamed water, scents, and the ability to touch.

The most important element of a sensuous bathing experience is the ability to indulge and having the time to do it. It is the ultimate cleaning pleasure. It has been the same since people flocked to public steam baths in ancient Sparta. Bathing helps humans care for their bodies. The rituals of bath treatments help unify mind, body, and spirit for overall well-being and cleaning. Today bathing increasingly benefits active and inquisitive lifestyles. Bathing is popular because it restores the body, balances life, revives the mind, and energizes the spirit.

BATHING TO MOISTURIZE

Women can find body treatments everywhere, from chair massages in grocery stores to full-day pampering at luxury spas. Women should apply a moisturizer treatment each night before falling asleep. She can start by telling everyone that she would like some privacy and relaxation, and then go to her room and start her moisturizing hygiene regimen.

She will need music, moisturizer, scented candles, a bathtub, and a fluffy bath towel. Then she should:

❧ Run a warm bath and add a favorite spritz, bath oil, cologne, or fragrance. While the water is filling in the tub, she can rub her body down with a favorite before-the-bath moisturizer and read her *Keeping the Home Fires Burning* book.

❧ Play her favorite music selection.

- ❦ Light a few small scented candles, turn the lights off, and ease into the freshly filled tub of water. Allow the water to envelope her awaiting body.

- ❦ Relax completely, physically and mentally. Allow the light of the candles to dance in her mind as it flickers her into an intensely mellow mood.

- ❦ The mood should guide her toward relaxation, enhancing her senses as she thinks of nothing but relaxation and sensual pleasures.

- ❦ Allow the quiet surroundings to swallow her as the scents entice her. Let the mood romance her desires as she humbles her soul to the pleasures of it all.

- ❦ Pull a handful of water toward her and feel the water as it trickles down her chest, between her breasts, and across her neck.

- ❦ Now unwind and let the senses lock in. That should feel good to her!

- ❦ Close her eyes and listen to the music playing softly as she gathers her senses and adores the peacefulness that surrounds her. Discover the serenity as the ripples of water disappear. Get lost in thought, and when she begins to feel drowsy, she may remove her new self from the tub. Pat dry with a fluffy towel and lightly moisturize again.

- ❦ Ease into bed and drift off to sleep. Sweet dreams.

AFTER BATHING

Every woman's body is unique, and no matter what kind of body she has, she is special. She will love experimenting with what makes her feel pampered.

She will need a bath towel, scented candles, lotion, oil, or moisturizer. Then she proceeds as follows:

- After a soothing bath, use a towel to dry off very slowly. With every stroke of the towel, blot gently as if drying off a newborn baby.

- Slowly massage the body with lotion, oil, or moisturizer. Try not to miss any areas.

- Applying lotions by candlelight is very soothing and romantic.

- Begin a my-body friendship. Know where every bump, scar, and mole are.

- Rub on any remaining lotion, pull the bed covers back, and ease into bed while naked.

- Think good thoughts about the skin she is in.

- Blow out the candles.

- In a short while, fall asleep. Sweet dreams.

A MAN'S BIGGEST COMPLAINT ABOUT HER HYGIENE

The biggest complaint from men about women who have a vaginal odor is that her vagina smells like onions or it tastes like urine. This leads me to believe that women need to clean better and wipe their vaginal area better after urination.

"When I'm good, I'm very good. But when I'm bad, I'm better.

~Mae West

Chapter 5

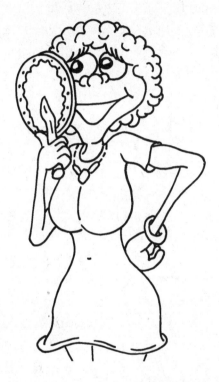

Her Appearance

She will never get into a man's heart or head unless she is pleasantly attractive and interesting. Even if she is not trying to please a man, she should at least be trying to improve herself.

A woman is a beautiful product, and she should be promoted. She should make sure she is packaged in the most positive way. It is beneficial to keep her personal appearance up to par. She does not have to be a beauty queen, but she should at least have a pleasing personal appearance.

She will never get into a man's heart or head unless she is pleasantly attractive and interesting to him. Even if she is not trying to please a man, she should always work to improve herself. She should not fret; all women have areas that need work or improvement. If she finds a need to improve certain areas, she should begin as soon as possible, working to create a new and healthy attitude about her appearance and personality.

HER PRESENTATION IS ESSENTIAL

She should wear her best underwear and never, ever be caught with dirty underwear or underwear held together by safety pins. Wearing bras held together by safety pins is one of the worst things a woman can do. She should invest in new undergarments and throw the old ones away. In the past, her parents encouraged her to always wear clean underwear in case she was in an accident and had to go to the hospital. She was instructed to take a bath, whether she needed it or not. Bathing fulfilled the main requirements of cleanliness. Today, requirements are stricter.

> **She Should Know**
>
> Every woman has a favorite set of sexy underwear whether she's sporty, girly, or tomboyish. She loves women's lingerie that makes her feel frilly, sweet, sexy, beautiful, daring, and so on. She loves bringing out her softer, wilder, sexier side.

Very brief, thin underwear looks good on both men and women. The more sensuous the undies, the more inviting they are. Since women and sex have become America's favorite pastime, personal care and grooming have become a national symbol of wholesomeness.

Television and radio commercials, movies, reality TV, and talk show hosts are now advertising flavored edible underwear. Our society cannot help but think about a woman's basic hygiene. A woman should think like that too.

HER FASHION CONSCIOUSNESS

A woman should evaluate herself and recognize her faults, paying close attention to areas that need extra work or attention. If she thinks these areas need extra work, then they probably do.

Collecting fashion magazines, articles, and pictures will help her coordinate new ideas for her existing wardrobe. By devoting some time and effort to her appearance on a regular basis, she will be able to find flattering clothes that complement her finer points. Seeing an improved "her" takes concentrated effort.

> **She Should Do**
>
> Good fashion sense starts with her personality. Ideally, her choice in fashion should express something about who she is as a person. She should jot down a list of personality traits and passions she would like to see conveyed by her wardrobe.

Another way to enhance her appearance or flatter her figure is to go to department stores, boutiques, or even discount stores with a friend to try on new kinds of clothing that she has always wondered what she would look like in. To minimize her figure faults, she should work with her good points. She should be fashion conscious and dress for success, but should not let fashion enslave her.

She should be a trendsetter; when everyone is wearing baggy pants and loose blouses, she chooses to wear slightly tight pants and a skimpy blouse. Most men are attracted to certain colors that women wear. In a survey of one hundred men, 70 percent chose blue as their favorite color. So, wear plenty of blue accents.

HER ANGLES

When wearing clothes, she should observe herself in the mirror from all angles—sitting, standing, squatting, and bending. To observe her strengths and weaknesses, she should check the following items:

- Does her clothing lie smooth or slide up?

- Is clothing maintenance easy or difficult?

- Does the skirt hike up in the back or front?

- How clean is the look?

- Is her skin smooth and beautiful?

- Do her teeth have stains and discolorations?

- Is her hair clean, fresh, and manageable looking?

- Are her ears and nose free from unsightly hair?

- Are her eyebrows evenly shaped?

- Is her makeup even and beautiful?

- Are her hands rough and harsh looking?

- Are her nails chipped and in need of a manicure?

- Are her shoes scuffed or scarred, run over, or dirty?

- Do her clothes appear dingy, rumpled, or faded?

- Do her clothes fit too tightly, or are they obviously too big?

A woman should feel good about incorporating these things. If she does, she can start working to improve today. She should be aware of her weaknesses; men certainly will.

HER NEATNESS

Even if she is a little on the wild side, a punk-rock type, or a mild, meek-mannered person, a woman should still be neat, clean, and attractive in her appearance: no runs in her hosiery, no holes in her socks, no faded fake earrings, no runny mascara, no smudges in her makeup, no smeared or uneven lipstick, no tacky eyebrows, no clumpy eyelashes, no scuffed handbags, no missing buttons, no broken zippers, and no dangling threads. And she should never wear day-old makeup. She should freshen up and remove old makeup from the skin on a daily basis, and touch up makeup as needed. She should check her clothing from top to bottom to make sure she is put together in the best way possible.

HER SHOES

When wearing shoes, flats should be worn in a woman's true foot size, but heels should be at least a half-size larger for comfort. This method eliminates corns and calluses, which are not a pretty sight on a woman. Shoes worn by a woman should convey a sense of purity and cleanliness. Shoes that are worn frequently should be made of leather or woven fabric. These materials breathe and are usually more comfortable than shoes made of synthetic materials.

A woman should wear shoes that complement her feet. A friend might wear sling backs because of the size and shape of her foot, but she might not be able to. Her shoe wardrobe should include a pair of shoes in a neutral color that go well with a wide range of clothing. She must be selective and complementary. When selecting or wearing shoes, she makes sure they are:

- Clean and shining
- Neat and fitting
- Never too tight or too small
- Polished, even, and free of any scuffmarks

SEDUCTIVE HEELS THAT APPEAL

Women have their own interpretation of how to wear heels seductively. Heels are a woman's pedestal, and she wears them as a sensual statement. High heels entice some men because of the sexuality they reveal. Heels give a woman's legs curve, elegance, and sexiness. Women with long legs create dramatic effects when donning a pair of heels. On women with short legs, heels can create length, which gives added height, and her heels can be as seductive as she wants.

HER BOOBS

It is obvious that men admire a woman's breasts, hips, butt, legs, arms, necks, and so on. Perhaps her attributes came from her family gene pool…like mama, like daughter. This is an area where style, size, and shape are subjective. The right bra on beautiful breasts can make a man's tongue drop to the floor. Bras with cotton straps are perfect for accentuating large boobs, and they keep the breasts steady.

Body and Soul

Boobs and butts are two of the most attractive and eye-catching female assets—so it's important to keep them both looking perky.

HER HANDS AND NAILS

A woman should focus on the little things when it comes to hands. As far as the hands are concerned, the minor things can quickly become major. When extending her hand, a woman must make sure it is a hand that others will want to hold. Hands are the final addition of a welcoming touch.

Beautiful nails are a plus. Clean, neat, and smooth-textured nails help a woman feel good about herself. Attractive nails speak to the time and attention she pays to herself. It is important for her to keep finger-nails and toenails manicured and polished, even if it is only a clear coat of polish. Even if no polish is needed, she should make it a habit to clean under the nails and trim unwanted cuticles or apply cuticle cream to soften the look. When it comes to polish, she should choose colors that complement her skin tone. Colors that look good on a friend may not compliment her. She should remain an individual by wearing what looks good on her.

When it comes to nail care, a woman should do the following:

- When nails chip excessively, it may be caused by excessive use of nail polish remover. She should leave nails unpainted for a few days to see if the condition improves.

- When preparing anything with lemon and vegetable juices, which contain acids that are hard on fingernails, she should rinse hands under cool running water.

- To break the habit of nail biting or cuticle chewing, she should carry a tube of cuticle cream. Whenever there's a desire to nibble, she can put the cream on cuticles. It promotes healthy nails and breaks a bad habit.

- To prevent polish from thickening, store it in the refrigerator.

- To rescue nail polish that has become hardened or gummy, place the bottle in a pan of boiling water for a few seconds to get the polish flowing smoothly again.

- Choose color carefully. A light color of nail polish gives hands the illusion of being longer and more graceful. Dark polish shortens fingers.

- Use an emery board to file nails in one direction.

- To prevent nail polish bottle tops from sticking, rubbing the inside of the cap and the neck of the bottle with a thin layer of petroleum jelly before closing works well.

HER HAIR STYLES

A woman should invest in a haircut or hairstyle that complements the beautiful features of her face. Not every hairstyle is presentable or intended to be worn by every face. She should be different, yet choose a style that is flattering. The basic cut is the key to an attractive hairstyle.

If the cut is not right, the style will not last, and it will not flatter the face, nor will it look fresh and neat on a daily basis.

If the hair looks too greasy, dull, or messy, all the beautiful designer clothing, perfectly applied makeup, and fine jewelry are wasted. Fortunately, no one needs an expensive professional hair salon or expensive hair products to have hair that looks professionally cared for and styled. With the right techniques for shampooing, drying, and styling, hair is one of a woman's most attractive features. The most obvious and effective way a woman can let a man know she is interested is to tousle her hair or stroke it continuously in his presence.

> **Watch Out**
>
> She should take a hot shower. For effective hair removal on any part of the body, pores need to be open. This can help reduce irritation of the skin. Soaking the hairs in warm or hot water also makes the hairs soften, resulting in safer hair removal.

SHAVING AND REMOVING UNWANTED HAIR

Hair under the arms or on the legs should be sheared. And if a woman has a mustache that keeps peeking out, get electrolysis if needed. As far as the rest of body hair, it is up to the woman whether she trims or shaves it.

A woman need not get carried away with trying to remove any hair, other than underarm and leg hair and obvious pubic hairs. Trying to shave the hair surrounding the navel or the hair on the nipples is unnecessary. Shaving hair in these places makes it comes back in triplicate, and the new growth is coarse and unattractive. She should be consistent about whatever hair she decides to remove, and remain conscientious about unsightly hair. Women tend to become very relaxed about such things when they are involved in a long-term relationship. This is being personally inconsiderate. The abrasive stubble can ruin a once-beautiful sensuous encounter.

HER GENITAL HAIR GROOMING

Hair in the genital area holds sweat and odor. Pubic hair is trimmed to keep unwanted odors to a minimum. A woman must trim or shave any long hairs that peek out from panties. It is unattractive and barbaric for a woman to present hairs hanging out of her underwear. Many men and women find that if the genital region of their lover is shaven, it's extremely erotic. On men, the removal of the pubic hair can make the male identity seem more vulnerable and much larger, which is a real turn-on for women. For couples who are interested in shaving, talk to each other about making it a fun activity that can be shared. If a woman chooses to shave her pubic region, she should:

- Trim long pubic hairs with clippers or scissors before using a razor to shave in close. Electric clippers are best for this.

- Take a very long, warm bath beforehand.

- Before applying shaving cream, rinse the area with cool water.

- Apply shaving cream a few minutes before shaving to soften hairs. Consider using shaving cream with additional conditioners or aloe.

- Use a sharp blade or two new blades if shaving a large area.

- Stroke an area no more than twice to reduce skin irritation. On the first stroke, go "with the grain" to remove most of the hair and then go "against the grain" for a smooth, close shave. If going against the grain irritates, then skip that and use both strokes with the grain.

- Clean the area afterwards with soap and water to reduce the risk of infection. Give the area a second cleansing using cotton balls and aloe.

- If irritations come from shaving, avoid shaving or try hypoallergenic shaving creams.

- If skin is sensitive, avoid shaving. Consider closely trimming the hair instead.

🌸 Letting hair grow out after shaving the pubic area can be a bothersome task. The sharp hairs combined with the sensitive skin will remind a woman how much movement happens in that area on an average day. Chafing is nearly unavoidable.

🌸 Talk to her lover about arranging to shave each other. This is a very erotic and sensual activity. Be sure to communicate clearly and proceed slowly. Find out what he likes, what feels good and what doesn't feel good.

🌸 Go as long as possible between shavings to reduce skin irritation. Happy shaving!

SHAMPOOING HER HAIR

If a woman would rather shampoo her own hair, she should check with her local pharmacist or hairstylist on which product or brand is best for her hair type. After shampooing, she rinses the hair with cool water to seal in the moisture in the hair shafts. For beautiful hair, she should try these tips:

🌸 To distribute the natural oils in the hair, bend over and brush the scalp and hair from back to front until the scalp tingles; then massage the scalp with fingertips.

🌸 If there is dandruff, use a good dandruff shampoo. Try the following treatment every two weeks: Section the hair and rub the scalp with a cotton pad saturated with plain rubbing alcohol. Let the alcohol dry; then brush the hair and rinse thoroughly with warm water, but do not shampoo.

🌸 To cut down on static electricity, slightly dampen the hairbrush before brushing hair.

🌸 Avoid using a brush on wet hair, because it is subject to breakage.

🌸 To get a fuller hairstyle, bend over and let hair fall forward and blow underneath layers.

- To perk up curly or permed hair between shampoos, lightly mist hair with fresh water and push the curls into place with fingers.

- Dull, lifeless hair is a sign of a poor diet. Try cutting down on cholesterol and fats.

- For colored hair: wait at least forty-eight hours after coloring hair before shampooing it again. Every time hair is wet, it opens the cuticle; give hair time to seal in the color.

- Hair sprays, mousses, gels, and other styling aids build up over time, despite regular shampooing and rinsing. If this happens, buy a clarifier, which removes product buildup without stripping essential oils. Mixing one part vinegar with twenty parts water will make a homemade clarifier.

HER EYES ARE SPEAKING

Even though silent, a woman's eyes speak volumes. A woman loves using her eyes to communicate her feelings. Her eyes sending seductive looks or the classic "glancing away and then looking back to see if he's still watching" is a technique that all women employ. A hybrid of this is when she looks over her shoulder, smiles, and then walks away.

A woman should look at a man's eye movements when she is talking to him. If there is a break in eye contact, she should look at his lips or chest and slowly work her way back to his eyes. It lets him know that she is interested in him. Her eyes are the windows to her soul. They tell the world who she is. The spirit behind the eyes is only one of the many keys to

She Should Know

Eyes can be a powerful tool when it comes to seduction. There are several ways she can use her eyes to display attraction and get someone interested in her. Make initial eye contact and, from there, make the most of the sensual gazing.

unlocking sensuality. Using the eyes as a creative and seductive tool can produce some of the most pleasurable moments in a relationship.

HER GOOD SMILE SHINES THROUGH

A bright smile projects health and good grooming. It is beautiful, and a man will continue to look at her repeatedly! He wants to kiss her. A beautiful smile displays white, smooth teeth that fill up the area within the lips. The lips frame a great smile like a masterpiece of art. Sexual attraction causes the lips to fill with blood, enlarge, and turn red. Perhaps this is why red or hot pink lipstick is preferred.

HER CLEAN AND HEALTHY SKIN

No matter the color of the complexion, a woman should keep her skin clean, healthy, and smooth. Someone is always looking at her complexion, so she should revel in it by keeping it wholesome looking.

People do not see the color of a woman's skin; they see the condition of it. Are her lips satiny smooth, blemish free, and healthy looking? Does her skin look as if she's has been kissed by the glimmer of the sun? Does it have a beautiful glow? Is it rich with vitality and alive? Is it the kind of skin a man would want to touch, even though she reserves the impulse for a more appropriate time? That kind of skin is worth the time and effort.

A woman should exfoliate the skin at least twice a month to keep it clean and healthy looking. There are wonderful over-the-counter exfoliating products available in local stores. Taking care of the skin allows its finer properties to gleam. The skin is a bellwether to overall health. If the woman is not healthy, it will be reflected in her

She Should Know

Her skin changes as she ages, especially during puberty, and looking for products in the skin-care aisle at the drugstore can be confusing. There are so many options! Which should you choose? It is important to first determine your skin type.

complexion, but that does not mean she should neglect her skin if she is feeling fine. To clear up skin problems, she should follow these easy rules:

- Do not play with or pick pimples. Put notes on mirrors as a reminder.

- Do not touch or lean cheeks on the cradle of the phone. Particles of food or secretions from the face or mouth may be there.

- Drink water to flush out impurities.

- Never sleep with makeup. If she hates to sleep with a naked face, she can dust lightly with pressed powder and blush.

- Get at least eight hours of sleep per night.

- Clean with astringent after working out.

- Avoid laundry detergents with sodium lauryl sulfate (pimple-producing ingredient).

- Take ibuprofen when cysts pimples appear to reduce the inflammation.

- To calm facial redness, take ice breaks twice a day for two minutes. Place cold towels or towels with crushed ice gently against the face for several minutes each morning. It will revitalize the face and make it feel fresh and perky.

- Read all cosmetic labels. Avoid products containing isopropyl myristate, isopropyl palmitate, stearic acid, decylo-leate, mineral oil, lanolin, and fragrance.

- Avoid getting hairstyling products on the forehead.

- A surprising blemish fighter is good SEX.

- Sun does not dry zits; it damages follicles, making the breakout worse. Use sunblock.

- Do not apply fragrances or colognes to the face to avoid irritations.

- Wear moisturizing sunscreen outdoors, winter and summer. The sun's rays can burn even if the air feels cool. Sunlight reflected off water or the whiteness of snow is powerful.
- Use a high-protection lotion the first time skin is exposed to sun for more than fifteen minutes.
- Use sunscreen on the face and back of hands, because they too are exposed to the sun's rays.
- Allow skin a chance to breathe by going without makeup.
- Use a humidifier to lessen drying effects of indoor air on the skin.
- Take baths in the evening to avoid exposing the skin to the outdoor air.
- Darker skin can get skin cancer. DO NOT evade sun block because of race.

HER LIPS

Lips comes in all sizes, shapes, colors, and textures…full, thin, pouty, voluptuous, and so on. For beautiful lips, a woman should:

- Apply lipstick all over and then blot to keep lips going all day.
- Avoid getting lipstick on her teeth. To remove lipstick from teeth, pucker lips into an extreme "O." Cover the index finger with tissue, and put it into the mouth and then slowly twist out of the mouth, removing excess color.
- Achieve a pouty, sexy mouth by emphasizing the top lip by dabbing gloss in the center.
- Highlight the lips with a very light eye shadow that coordinates with lip color tones. Place it in the center of the upper and lower lips.
- Balance unevenly shaped lips by using a lighter colored lipstick on the smaller-sized lip.

❦ Take care to keep lipstick in place while dining by keeping the lips off utensils. Allow the lower teeth and tongue to do the work.

❦ Rub a washcloth over lips before applying lipstick to smooth lips.

HER FULL LIPS

Women who have large lips are lucky. Women everywhere try to replicate that look with collagen, but large lips can take over the face if a woman is not careful. To prevent this, she should do the following:

❦ For fuller-looking lips, line them and then blend the edges with a sponge applicator. Cover with gloss or petroleum jelly.

❦ To make full lips appear slimmer, draw a line inside the natural lip line and fill with a darker shade of lip color.

❦ Avoid lip liner; simply soften the edges with a Q-tip.

❦ Not wear any lip color that is too glossy or shiny. Full lips can begin to look more like a butt than lips

HER THIN LIPS

To make thin lips appear fuller, a woman should try these cosmetic tricks:

❦ Draw slightly beyond the lip with a neutral-colored lip pencil. Fill with a lighter shade of lipstick. Lipstick will catch onto the liner.

❦ Apply white shadow on center of lips over lipstick and spread slightly.

❦ Avoid very dark shades of lipstick, which make lips look small and dirty.

❦ Protect thin lips with a thin coating of colorless lip balm when not wearing lip color.

- For long-lasting lipstick, apply a generous coat and let it set for about two minutes. Blot with a tissue, put on some powder, and then apply another coat of lipstick. Wait again, and blot.

- Choose warm, tawny lip colors for office light.

- If lips are uneven, apply foundation over them and then fashion a new lip line with a pencil a shade darker than the lip color.

HER SEXY TEETH

Enlarged lips are less obvious as women get older because teeth wear down as the lips get thinner. As a result, there is less lip. Older, worn teeth are often the same length, but a youthful, sexy smile displays longer central incisors, slightly shorter laterals, and smooth, unworn cuspids. A beautiful smile takes the lines from the face, enlarges the lips, and shows more teeth. A beautiful, sexy smile displays the upper front teeth and hardly any of the lowers. Revealing too much gum is considered unattractive, but a fantastic smile boasts white teeth and beautiful gums.

HER ARMS ARE SEXUAL TOOLS

It is amazing how much we adore great-looking arms. Men notice them because they denote strength and firmness. They do not need to be muscular, but nicely toned arms are appealing to men. A woman's arms are made for embracing and holding on to the people she loves. Reaching with outstretched arms that are fit and toned is sexy on any woman.

HER SEXY NECK

A woman can use any part of her body to speak to a man, but negative comments are made daily about a woman having a neck with rolls of excess skin. When a woman has a smooth and sleek neck, she is rewarded with flattery. A taut, good-looking neck reflects youth, pride, well-being, and sexiness. A neck is a tender place to put lips on. Women perfume their necks and train their necks to tease the opposite sex.

A woman's neck portrays elegance grace, power, beauty, and prowess when she is working it from side to side.

HER SEXY LEGS

Men tend to observe how a woman positions her legs. It is hard to understand the exact scientific mechanics of how women flirt with their legs, but legs are highly visible and useful for turning men on. That is not by accident. It does not matter whether a woman's legs are long or short, skinny or thick—it is every man's dream to caress them. By finding the right dress, skirt, or shorts to complement the legs, she will strut with grace and elegance.

HER BEAUTIFUL FEET ARE SWEET

We all know at least one man who loves a woman's legs, but to find a man who loves feet is unique. Men may not touch feet often, but they sure do notice them. Are they clean and neatly manicured, or are they hard and callused, looking like she just participated in a marathon barefooted? Her feet indicate how much attention she pays to her overall grooming experience. Does she take the time to care for her feet? How well she takes care of her feet says a lot about her to a man. She should give honor to all parts of the body, especially the feet.

HER POSTURE AND POSITIONING

If a woman is interested in a man, her posture is very perky and poised when he is around. Her back is arched and her chest is slightly pushed forward. An interested woman will try to close the distance between her and the man she is interested in. If she is leaning into the man or standing closer than normal with a relaxed (almost inviting) stance, she is making herself approachable. However, if she is standing upright with arms crossed, she is not interested.

Her posture is important in her overall appearance and she can improve it by visiting any lingerie department and ask a fitter to size her properly so that her breasts will not sag or hang, and to ensure she is not fitted with a bra too small, too tight, or too large. Okay…chest up, stomach in, butt high!

HER FRAGRANCES, PERFUMES, COLOGNES

Aromas enhance women's sexual arousal, but men might be surprised at the scrumptious scents that keep a woman's fire lit. The road to romance is not doused with he-man cologne. Clean, fresh scents work better for women, and reports confirm that both sexes find some of the same fragrances exciting.

> **She Should Know**
>
> Rubbing petroleum-jelly-based ointments on pulse points before spraying perfume can make the scent last longer. The ointment is occlusive and will hold the fragrance to skin longer than if it were sprayed onto dry skin.

Odors can also be associated with either a happy or a sad memory. Fragrances that excite women are usually fresh-smelling or nostalgic reminders of childhood—perhaps eating candy in movie theaters, sniffing pies at family gatherings, or getting a whiff of freshly baked cookies. It may also bring back memories of safety and security that she felt when she was being held in her lover's arms.

Cherry fragrance might be a turnoff because the taste is connected mentally to medicine and cough drops taken during illness. The barbecue odor is a mystery, but avoiding it is not a bad idea if she is interested in arousal. Think about it: does she recognize the fragrances that are turn-ons, and can she identify the scents, odors, or fragrances that are turnoffs?

Unless she (or her man) has allergic reactions to perfumes, colognes, or fragrances, she should wear them. Cheap imitations are simply that: "cheap imitations." When a woman is complimented about or been asked the name of the perfume she is wearing, she should take it as well-deserved praise. If asked more than several times a day, it is usually a very good indication that she has hit on a good fragrance that complements her body chemistry. A woman should ask herself these questions about fragrance:

- "Am I wearing the fragrance for myself or other people?"
- "How often do I wear the fragrance?"
- "How does wearing fragrance make me feel?"
- "How many different fragrances do I own?"
- "When was the last time I purchased a new fragrance?"

GET THE MOST FROM FRAGRANCES

If she wants to get the most from a fragrance, it should be worn on all pulse spots of the body. Apply perfume and cologne on the skin, rather than on clothes. Chemicals in fragrances may weaken fabric or change its color. To maximize the power of a fragrance, a woman should:

- Dab lightly. Colognes may clash with other smells.
- Choose a fragrance that complements her natural body odor.
- Avoid mixing too many smells, such as deodorant, lotions, powders, and perfumes. All of them on the same body can be quite repulsive. Many companies make lotions, body oils, perfumes, soaps, and bath gels in the same scent to help women in choosing. Odorless deodorants are available too.

WHERE TO APPLY FRAGRANCES

Apply fragrance on these body parts several times a day.

- Ankles
- Palms
- Back of knees
- Bend of elbows
- Behind the ears
- Base of the throat

❦ Bosom

❦ Inside wrists

❦ Between thighs

Fragrance is seductive and gets a woman noticed, but a quick spritz is not the only way to go. To make a definite and lasting impression, a woman can try these simple techniques:

1. Twirl! Spray fragrance in the air and spin in the mist. The misty molecules of spray should settle on her awaiting body, hair, and clothing …yummy.

2. Lightly scent a cotton ball or a hankie and stuff it in her bra, pocket, or glove.

3. Re-scent. Just as she would touch up her lipstick, she should touch up her fragrance. This combats fade-out and olfactory overload because her nose does not register odor once she has become used it.

4. If she cannot afford the real thing, less expensive bath oils and moisturizing lotions are potent and REALLY last! Dab as she would with perfume.

5. Check out new eau de parfum. They fall between toilet water and perfume in strength but are much less expensive.

6. Use matching bath and body products to layer fragrances.

7. Multifloral and oriental scents stay vital the longest and are arousing.

8. Avoid buying a scent just prior to menstruation, when sense of smell is weakest. (The birth control pill is said to also alter odor-detecting ability.)

9. Mix a few drops of perfume with conditioner and then run it through the hair. Hair is a fabulous perfume vehicle.

10. The best time to apply fragrances is after a shower, when pores soak up the aroma.

11. Dab petroleum jelly on pulse points and then apply perfume to these areas.

12. Apply perfume and cologne before putting on jewelry. The alcohol and oils in scents can cause a cloudy film on both real gold and costume jewelry.

13. Do not stick to one fragrance all year long. Temperatures affect the intensity of fragrance. Use heavy scents and oils in winter but light fragrances in small quantities in the summer.

USING FRAGRANCE TO IMPROVE HER SENSUALITY

A woman is equipped with sensuous tools, but to achieve great levels of sexuality she should learn how to use her tools. There are things a woman should know and understand about what it takes to become sensuously turned on. Perfume is a great motivator; however, if fragrance causes a bad reaction or abrasions appear, it will make life a living hell. So, use caution.

GUIDELINES BEFORE READING FURTHER

- A woman should consult a gynecologist before trying any suggestions in this book.

- She should read and discuss the chapters before attempting any of the suggestions.

Good sex awakens sexuality and defuses sexual tension.

Chapter 6

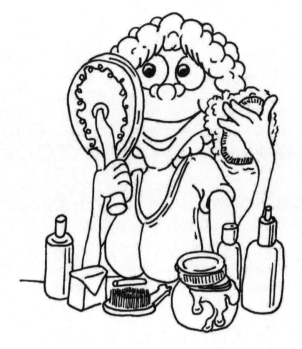

Her Sexual Radiance

She embraces her sexuality by embracing her inner vixen.

We have all seen that woman whose face and body would never grace the cover of a fashion magazine, yet all eyes follow her when she enters the room. She is positively noticed because her radiance attracts attention. Her walk exudes confidence, and she radiates with positive energy. Everything about her says, "I'm hot, I'm desirable, I'm sexy—and I know it." She is the woman who feels comfortable in her own skin, and her actions show that she is confident with her sexuality. We all know that this kind of self-confidence is great for any woman's ego. Everyone who meets and greets her wants to be around her.

Men confess that they admire a confident woman. When a woman is confident in

> **She Should Know**
>
> A self-assured woman not only admits her imperfections, but applauds them. She knows where her strengths lie, where she can improve, and when to get the heck outta dodge and let others take the lead. Trying to be perfect at everything is inefficient, and a confident woman does not have time for that. She loves herself for who she is—and for who she is not.

herself, she is sexier to men. When a woman has inner confidence and displays it, she has an inner beauty that shines outward.

HER SEXUAL CONFIDENCE

The best way for her to become sexually confident is to believe she is deserving of pleasures. She embraces her sexuality by embracing her inner vixen. All it takes is an attitude change. Instead of wondering if she is sexy, she knows that she is. For any woman to become sexually confident, she can:

1. Indulge in private self-pleasuring. Do not be afraid. When a woman understands how her body feels, she explores self-love. It helps her understand what she likes and how she likes it. No one else has to know.

2. Get to know her body. Know it better than any man ever could. She should not allow a man to touch her body before she is familiar with her own body. She should know what she likes and dislikes when her body is touched.

3. Dress sexy. Do not wait for a special occasion. Dress up, just because. Get rid of dingy, torn, beat-up, and faded clothing. She can dress up because she feels good about herself.

4. Invest in sexy underwear. She can visit a lingerie store and buy the sexiest underwear that will fit. Put it on. She should notice how sexy she feels. Now she can wear sexy underwear under everyday clothing for no reason. Wear it, just because.

5. Bring sexy back! Radiate with sexiness. When she knows she is sexy, she can feel sexy. If she feels sexy, she will radiate sexiness.

6. Remember the great saying: "You are what you feel." It is true. Sometimes a woman might not feel sexy, but the moment she begins to think and believe she is, people around her will begin to think that she is. It is amazing how much a woman's sexiness begins to blossom when she feels it. Sexiness begins in the mind. For the most part, it is all mental. Possess sexual confidence. The most positive thing a woman can do for her self-esteem is learn what to do and how to act. She should learn to present herself in a way that improves her confidence level. The most beautiful woman becomes more graceful and charming when she radiates self-esteem. Women who communicate with confidence often display sassy feminine assets in a positive way and are more appealing to men.

7. Concentrate on him. A woman who takes pride in making her lover feel good in bed knows that in order for her to get his attention she has to find his libido. Taking a few tips from the female pros is not a bad idea either. Focus the attention on his face, ears, skin, arms, legs, chest, and the rest of him. Get so involved in him that he feels like he is the only person in the world. He should feel that she is mesmerized by his presence.

8. Do sexy things. She should notice when he touches her and the way he does it, and then later reverse the touching so that he enjoys it just as much as she does. If he strokes her between the thighs and it gives her chills, she should do the same to him

later. If he likes to suck on her fingers, she should do the same to him. A man enjoys a woman who does sexy things to him.

9. Avoid negative people, things, and situations. Replace them with positive and empowering messages. Any negative messages received in the past can be replaced with encouraging messages. If her partner says hurtful things to her, she should get rid of him and move on to a positive person.

10. Adopt a positive attitude about life. Life is too short to let the good pass. Begin today by opening her heart and mind to new experiences.

11. Begin the day with "I love me because _____." It makes her feel better for the rest of the day.

12. Indulge in nakedness. When getting out of the tub, do not be so quick to put on clothes. Walk around naked for at least fifteen minutes.

13. Write her life story with her as the main character. Initiate sex tonight. Be open to making the first move. Go ahead—what is there to lose?

14. Study sex manuals. Open up and accept positive love.

15. Create a romantic atmosphere. Buy sensuous candles, sexy clothing, and plush bed covers, and indulge in stimulating foods.

But beauty itself is not given to us by anyone; it is a power we have within us from the gate, a radiance inside us.

~Marianne Williamson

Chapter 7

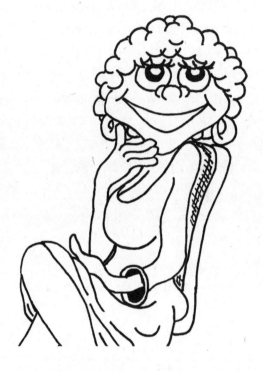

Her Mental Foreplay

A woman's imagination is the sexiest turn-on of all.
Giving her lover something to think about will make him sensuously hard in
all the right places.

Since the brain is the most erotic part of the body, how and what a woman thinks sets the tone for sensuous moments. What encourages her to feel and act sexy when she is with her lover? Are those delicious thoughts of being romantic, touching, feeling, tasting, and of course making sensuous love?

What does it take to get sexually motivated and excited? What sexually satisfies her? Does kissing her man turn her on? Does rubbing certain parts of his body against hers excite her? Do the thoughts of sensuous penetration move her into a sexual zone? What does he do that makes her squirm thinking of it? What wonderful things bring her to great levels of sensual excitement? Can she say the things that get him in the mood and be halfway there? A man gets turned on thinking about how she looked the last time he saw her. Her imagination is the sexiest turn-on of all. Giving him something to think about will get him hard in all the right places. When she combines sex and imagination she can reap sensuous rewards if she:

1. Tell her lover about the big and small things that are a sure turn-on.

2. Share erotic pictures with him. Men love pictures of women doing erotic things.

3. Open up the lines of communication by telling him there is something he should see and then present him with several erotic magazines. He will love it.

4. Share sensuous pictures with him. If there are none to be found, she can take some sexy photos. Use an instant camera so no one else will see them.

5. Read erotic paragraphs from *Keeping the Home Fires Burning*. Read with the goal of turning him on.

6. Greet him at the door dressed in a maid's costume: a tiny cap, high heels, a small black apron, and sexy hosiery.

7. Make a tape of his sounds during a sexual act. Listen to the tape, and if it needs to be re-taped, happily redo it. Sounds of lovemaking will have him wanting to make love again.

8. Write him a sensuous poem and slip it into his wallet. He will be warmly surprised.

9. While together in a restaurant, waiting in line, or visiting friends, look in his eyes and whisper to him what pleasures are in store for him. Be specific, smile, and then change the subject.

10. Buy sexy clothing to wear for him. Model it for him.

11. Send pieces of lingerie in the mail. Enclose a note describing what pleasures await him later.

She is deserving of pleasure, and
pleasure is best when it is embraced.

Chapter 8

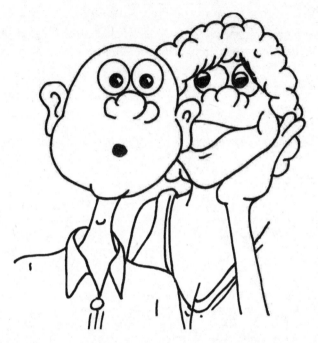

Her Sensual Conversations

What a wonderful rush that travels up and down his spine when his lover is saying the things he likes to hear.

Women love conversations that are not forced upon them. They might tease and play with the words, enjoying not getting to the point right away. Sex is a sensitive conversation that is not always easy for women to talk about, especially when the conversation might include sex games, toys, and sexual interludes. Because bad people have given good sex a sour reputation, it's important to communicate the positive side of intimacy and sexuality of consenting adult women. I will hide nothing from women.

Women are grateful when they learn this information, and as they learn, they begin to experience confidence that brings happiness in and out of their bedrooms. Frankly, they smile more, are more relaxed, and have less frustration when they are sensuously in tune with their sexual wants, needs, and desires. When women are sexually fulfilled, they are happy, and their personal relationships embody this same happiness.

> **She Should Know**
>
> Some women do not feel dependent on their partner for the expression of their sexuality.

Conversations consist of not only what is said, but also how it is said. The more accomplished a woman's conversation is, the more she can use her voice tone, facial expressions, and gestures for emphasis, thought, wit, and empathy when conversing.

Conversations that involve sensuous talk are delicious. What a wonderful rush that travels up and down a woman's spine when her lover is saying the things she likes to hear. Her brain takes what he says and thinks what the words will be like when turned into actions. Women are turned on by sensuous verbal fantasy.

Sensuous conversation is not simply an exclamation of moans, groans, and squeals until finally—ejaculation. Erotic turn-ons can be interpreted in several different ways. The best turn-ons are in the ears of the receiver. An erotic turn-on is one of the most potent means for changing direct and sensuous talk into an inviting verbal adventure.

HER SOUNDS OF ECSTASY

Noise is associated with sex whether the sex is good, bad, pleasurable, or painful. She might feel inhibited or even foolish when being verbal during lovemaking because of its unfeminine like characteristics. Women sometimes do not want men to recognize the fact that they are enjoying themselves. If a woman wants sounds to be a natural part of her sexual pleasure, she should verbally express it. As she becomes aroused, her heart rate and breathing speed up. As she begins to reach orgasm, it speeds up three to four times faster than normal. No sensuous woman can keep still when all this noise and excitement are going on. Men are turned on by a woman's sounds of ecstasy. It makes him feel like the king of her night, but there are still some men who feel noise is a turnoff or distracting.

> **She Should Know**
>
> A sexually confident woman doesn't dim her light so that everyone will like her. Instead, she shines brightly so that everyone can see her.

Exposure to sex talk is rewarding and quite an experience if it is with someone she loves and adores. The biggest complaint is that sex talk makes some women feel cheap and dirty. Then there are women who love sex talk and everything about it. Some women are so into it that they script what they want their lovers to say to them.

HER RELAXATION

Relaxing and going with the flow is a positive thing when she is with the man she loves. A woman will shortly find herself being turned on by sex talk in a sensuous way if she thinks about it positively. For example, if he says, "Suck me, baby," then she will say to him, "I love the way you turn me on." Then, one night when making love, she should get immersed in the sensuous thought of it all and let private thoughts become a matter of verbal arousal. After doing this a few times, she will look forward to it. Verbal arousal takes practice at first. After a few times it becomes very natural to indulge in it.

If sex talk is too difficult, she can seductively verbalize her feelings by saying simple things like, "Ummmmm, I like that," or "Ummmmm, I needed that." It will give her the practice she needs without talking dirty. As she accepts and receives love, she can practice verbalizing her desires and feelings, so that she can communicate with her lover in an erotic way.

Another great way to start verbalizing is to tell him what she wants

> **She Should Know**
>
> She's not afraid of being the center of attention. She's confident in who she is and what she has to offer the world.

and if it feels good during love-making. Saying things that make him feel good or making sexual requests while making love is a great way to let her guard down and start verbalizing. He will love her for it.

HER SOOTHING VOICE

While making love, nothing is more erosive to a man than a woman who has an irritating voice. No man wants to hear a scratchy voice when he is holding her in the heat of passion. A woman can practice improving her voice by listening to it on a tape recorder. She should not sound like she has laryngitis. That is unsexy and unromantic. It would be a shame to spend so much time and money looking beautiful only to have him be turned off hearing her voice. She should try the following voice-improvement techniques:

- ❦ Take a deep breath and hold for approximately five to eight seconds before answering the phone. Release and then breathe slowly while speaking. This adds to the sensuality of the voice. Continue practicing this technique until it is natural, fluent, and pleasant.

- ❦ Soften the tone with a lower voice. Women who have loud and boisterous voices are a turnoff.

- ❦ Practice pronunciation and correct word usage. Women with beautiful speaking voices and good pronunciation are double forces of seductiveness.

Words that begin with the letter *s* encourage provocative sounds. I have listed a few: suck, sucked, sucking, sex, sexy, sensuous, sensual, sequence, seduction, seep, semaphore. To find sensuous *s* words, she should look in the index of this book. Reciting *s* words build a sensuous vocabulary. But words beginning with *sh* are not sexy.

A woman should use the speech organs to produce provocative sounds when speaking. If she is willing to put forth the effort, a sweet, soft, sexy voice will lure any willing man in her direction. The truth is, men want to feel needed, and they need to be wanted. It is up to the woman to make a man feel needed, just as it is his responsibility to make her feel needed. Imagine all that she can accomplish when she says the right things in the right way in the correct tone.

HER SELF-EXPRESSION

It is not what a woman says as much as how she says it. The flavor of her language is part of her personality and feminine appeal. Some women use baby talk when communicating intimately with their lover. Anna Nicole Smith was famous for using baby talk when she wanted to receive affection. Some women use foreign language, and some moan and groan passionately. She does not have to do it all at once; she can gradually work her way into it. She can slowly express herself.

How does she express herself in her everyday situations? Is she funny, witty, straight to the point, or clever? Does she jump from one subject to the next? Has she pinpointed the type of talk she emanates, and can she translate that same formula to her sensual needs and desires?

HER TELEPHONE SAVVY

Phone sex is a wonderful way to encourage the most brilliant fantasies. No one can see her, so a woman can feel safe. It is almost like being alone, but expressing her deepest fantasies. Giving good phone sex is great for keeping the relationship steamy. She can use her sexy voice to make a man feel good and build his ego. A woman's ability to be perceptive on the phone will keep any man interested. She can seduce him by calling him and saying erotic things. She should assure him he is missed and then tell him he will not regret her pleasures. Some other obvious reasons for phone sex are:

1. There is no need to dress for the occasion.

2. Threats of unsafe sex are not present.

3. Phone sex is nonthreatening to the listener because face-to-face rejection does not exist.

4. There is always someone to talk with.

5. People engaging in phone sex can use their imagination without embarrassment.

6. Experiencing phone sex can teach her many aspects of sexuality that she has never thought about before. Exaggeration is natural on the telephone.

There are professional phone sex lines, but this section will deal with a woman's personal phone as a means of having phone sex with her lover.

HER ATTITUDE IS IMPORTANT

A woman's overall attitude is very important. To turn him on with phone sex, she should at least sound like a person who is genuinely interested in the phone conversation. While talking to him, she should use vivid adjectives that describe a favorite pleasurable encounter. If she has not had the pleasure of a sexual encounter but she wants one, she should describe what she would like to do to him. The description she provides should help her man create a pleasurable image in his mind.

> **She Should Know**
>
> She's comfortable in her own skin and knows that being authentic to her true self is the only way to be.

HER SEXIEST-SOUNDING VOICE

A good point for a woman to remember about voice quality is to think, act, and talk sensuously. If a woman believes in her sensuality, she will become the sensuous person she has always wanted to be. She must practice speaking clearly and make sure her voice is not abrasive or harsh. She should choose words that provoke sexy sounds. She can practice by using a hushed-low, sexy voice and making sounds of pleasure that give vivid images to her partner. Making love over the phone usually lasts longer than it does in real life. But a woman must not fall into the trap of using the phone as a way to avoid pleasure or a real relationship. Phone sex is for entertainment and not a replacement for kissing, cuddling, or a real beating heart. Here are some pointers a woman can use to help pull out her best and sexiest voice from within:

- Listen to her sexiest voice with a cassette.
- Learn what works. Call a phone sex line and learn the do's and don'ts of phone sex.
- Remain mentally seductive by having a gentle introduction.
- Have a slow buildup and soft resolution.
- Create a pet name that she can use in the dark.
- Choose his favorite song as the background music. Make sure it is seductive and low, and relates to both partners.
- Choose a long-playing song that makes the moment feel romantic.
- Choose a comfortable environment where she won't be interrupted.
- Turn the ringer off on the phone.
- Try not to sound rehearsed.
- Use his name or the nickname she gave him.
- Tell him what sexy thoughts she has had about the two of them.

- ❧ Choose sexy clothing, then take it off and go naked. It heightens the sensuality.

- ❧ While masturbating, tell him what she is doing as she does it.

- ❧ Be as honest as possible. Intently intensify…no faking.

- ❧ Rest for at least an hour after the tape is complete, and then listen to it. If she decides to mail it to him, send an erotic note with it. One-day mail services are quite nice.

- ❧ Put the tape in his lunch box or slip it in his car.

If she breathes when she talks, her voice will sound sexier.

PART 3

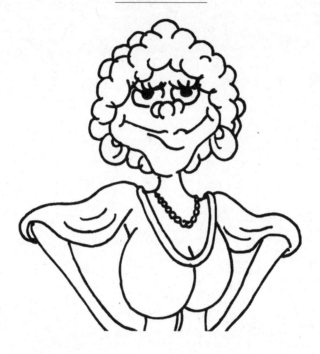

How to Improve Her Sensuality

Chapter 9

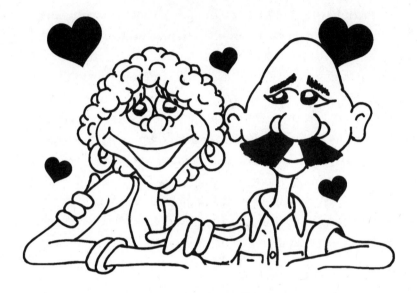

Her Touch

Touching promotes a healthy mind, body, and soul.
It calms us down and relieves our stress.

We have heard so much about the power of touch that it is taken for granted. Physical touch is so powerful it can sway the opinion of the opposite sex. All of us—young and old, single or in a relationship—need to be touched. The act of touching communicates more than words. Physical contact is a prerequisite for a healthy individual and for a fulfilling, mature, loving relationship.

Our bodies require touch; it relieves stress and makes us happier and healthier. In our fast-paced lives, we often forget the importance of giving and receiving affection through physical touch. We deprive ourselves of this very basic need, and we often deprive our loved ones. I cannot emphasize enough how important touch is in any loving relationship. We strive to diet, to quit smoking, to drink in moderation, and to exercise in order to promote a healthy body. However, touching is the most vital gift for health that a woman can give and receive.

Touching promotes a healthy mind, body, and soul. Touching calms us down, it relieves our stress, and it allows us to demonstrate our love for one another. If she has young children, when a woman arrives home they are excited to see her, and they will want physical contact from her. They want a hug, a cuddle, and a kiss. It makes them feel loved and cared for, and gives them the security that they need from her. After a long, stressful day, a hug and cuddle from her child, her partner, or even a friend are the best medicine she can get and give.

TOUCHING AS PART OF HER PLEASURE

The most basic form of sexual pleasure begins with a touch. A woman becomes familiar with her pleasures through touch. Does she know where she wants to be touched? Does she know how she likes to be touched? Knowing what she likes is the key to achieving her very own sexual satisfaction. Getting in touch with her body and her sexuality helps a woman get in tune with her emotional needs. She likes it when her lover touches her and when she is touching herself.

EVEN SINGLES NEED TOUCHING

She might be single at this time, but being single does not mean that she will not need touch and physical closeness in her daily life, especially if she has recently ended a relationship. As a single woman, she might be missing the hugs, kisses, embraces, and hand-holding that she once had. Her life and the world do not stop because she is not in a loving relationship—neither does her need for physical closeness and touching. It all starts within. The art of touching encompasses nonsexual and sexual touch, and it's important to get her daily allowance of it. Demonstrating physical closeness with family and friends is one way to elevate the mood, allowing her to feel loved and fulfilled, while giving love to others. This type of touching does wonders for a woman's health.

> **She Should Know**
>
> A sexually confident woman doesn't think that being a woman makes her *less than*. Instead, she sees her femininity as a gift.

Receiving a massage, manicure, pedicure, or even a haircut can provide the touching and physical stimulation that a woman needs. If she is in a relationship, both sexual and nonsexual touching is important. During the euphoric stage of a relationship, sexual touch predominates. She cannot keep her hands off him, nor can he keep his hands off her.

When mature love begins, nonsexual touch becomes more important, as touch takes on an additional meaning. While sexual touch can communicate sexual feelings, nonsexual touch can simply communicate love, care, and affection.

ENHANCING HER TOUCH

In a loving relationship, a woman should make a concerted effort to touch her partner. She should make sure that she and her partner do not forget to hug and kiss one another before leaving for work, or when returning home. They should take advantage of quiet moments during the day to give affectionate touching to one another. One simple example is to hold hands in a movie, at a restaurant, or while walking down the street. A woman's personal touch adds to a man's world and makes her unique in his eyes. Her touch is not just a beautifier; it is a stabilizer to men, children, pets, and ultimately the world at large.

> **She Should Know**
>
> Sensual touch can help her connect with her partner, show concern, receive affection, and relax.

We often forget the importance of touching our loved ones, our pets, others, and ourselves.

During intimate moments, people use sensuous touching more frequently. Touching enhances arousal and relays affection, sensitivity, and care. The pleasure of a sensitive touch keeps women connected to their partners from the first time they brush up against each other to the way they move in sync during intimate moments. Does she know that orgasms can be achieved through sensuous touching? When people are touching each other, they are not usually thinking about anything except that moment. They are thinking, *This feels soooo good—I want more.*

Sex is more alluring if touching is included before, during, and after sexual acts. Changing positions regularly while touching can improve the sex act. Sex feels different when the male identity is thrusting inside the vagina at different angles and a soothing touch accompanies it.

It feels great when different parts of the body are being touched at different intervals of sex. Figuring out what turns him on when touching at different times of the sexual act is quite exhilarating. For example, if a woman is having sex with the man on top, he can feel her breasts on his chest, her nipples rubbing against his skin, or her butt against his thighs.

Both sexes love touching, but men choose to admire the big picture whereas women love the small, involved moments that touch instills. Women are more in tune with their senses and seek the so-called pleasant surprises in everything they touch, smell, feel,

> **She Should Know**
>
> Sensual touch can be a great form of foreplay. However, it doesn't have to lead to genital touching at all. It can be very pleasurable in itself, and if she can't, or doesn't want to engage in sexual activity, this can be a great way to bond, relax, and have fun.

see, hear, and taste. Women love the idea of doing things that warm their heart. If a man can touch a woman's soul, he can transform her mood.

SENSUOUS TOUCHING

There are several pleasurable ways a woman is emotionally connected to her lover. First, she will need to take steps to get more in touch with her emotional side. To achieve rich, satisfying sex, every woman needs to take a journey of self-awareness. With such wonderful touching going on, she can discover sensuous ways to increase her sexual temperature. Besides, she and her lover will enjoy this private oasis. He will love getting stimulated while making love. Now that she has learned the magical powers of sensuous touching, she can rhythmically integrate touch and temperature into the relationship.

During sensuous touching time, a woman can enjoy the following exercises with her partner:

1. Try having sex without air conditioning on a hot day and enjoy the sweat rolling down the face, chest, and body.

2. Have a quickie in a hot tub at its steamiest moment.

3. Have sex on a cold winter day in the snow.

4. Play with ice cubes during sex and notice the difference.

5. Alternate sexual adventures with hot and cold fluids to give a variety of feelings to her lover.

6. Gently scratch him, tickle him, or soothe him by stroking his ears.

7. Alternate soft and hard objects with cold and hot touching.

8. With an oiled body, rub him up and down, side to side, and all over, body to body.

9. Shave body hair and allow him to feel the texture of the skin rubbing against his body.

10. Find soft fabrics or textures to slide against his body from time to time.

11. Experiment with sensuous touching in locations he's always wanted to have sex.

12. Have great sex on a cool day and experience the breeze blowing over his skin.

13. Have sex in the woods with the sounds of autumn while rolling in crackling leaves.

14. Have sex in the woods in the wintertime or during hot summer months and enjoy nature's scenes. Feel the warmth of the sun.

15. Have sex in the car against the glass windows as the car steams up.

16. Try giving pleasurable body massages without sex.

To give and get the best loving touches, a woman must know who she is, what she wants, and what she desires. When she knows what she wants, she can accept pleasurable touching in her life. It helps improve her sensuality.

Touching is a do-it-herself project.

Chapter 10

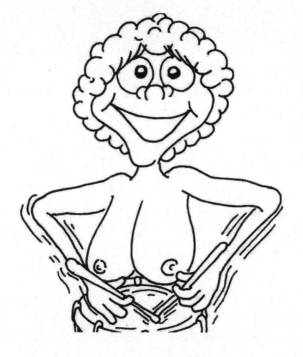

Her Sexual Rhythm!

She should evolve; make sexual music,
remembering that sex has a rhythm of its own.

Although women have tremendous sensual capacity, most never come close to realizing their sensual potential. They are trained to turn themselves off to much of what surrounds them. There are times that a woman has to slow down and feel what she is giving and receiving. During sex, women tend to like it slow; men like it faster. When a woman moves too fast, she can lose her sexual rhythm. She has to remember that her sex has a rhythm of its own.

All she has to do is open her arms, listen to her heart, close her eyes, and get in the right frame of mind. She should not ever lose her sexual balance. Slowing down, feeling the feeling, satisfying the soul, and easing the mind helps her to evolve. However, she has to create her own sexual rhythm with her lover. When they make love, they create their own unique rhythm.

FIND THE CURE FOR WHAT AILS HER RHYTHM

The rhythm of pleasure is great. Let us explore the example of a friend of mine who had lost her sexual edge due to years of emotional neglect from her partner.

My friend Marsha moved to Lewisville after living in Duncanville, Texas, with her husband, and found that she had to desensitize herself to his name-calling, lackluster behavior. In order to preserve her rhythm, she restricted her thoughts of what felt good and what was good in her life. The atmosphere in her home was an unhappy one, so much so that she placed positive Post-it notes in every room to maintain her sanity. Marsha had lost her rhythm. She decided that if she wanted to get her rhythm back she would have to make a change in her life.

She decided to use her ability to turn off things. This skill is helpful, particularly when dealing with situations that would otherwise be intolerable. She was able to turn off the critical or harmful comments received from an uncaring partner in order to deal with him or shield herself from his uncaring ways. She turned off sexually with her less-than-desirable partner. However, this easy process of turning off or turning on can become a pattern and will ultimately limit her ability to respond appropriately to new and better situations. Even when the source of anxiety is removed, the patterns are still there. The woman who shuts out a critical partner may turn into someone who is unable to feel anymore.

If a woman loses her rhythm, she has to find it again. She has to find her balance. She has to find her way. Simply put, she

> **Body and Soul**
>
> Discovering pleasurable places on her body can be super exciting, especially when done with someone who cares.

has to find her ability to love again. When it comes to developing her senses as it relates to sexual awareness, she is truly in double jeopardy. Women are encouraged to dress in the most provocative and expensive designer clothing but are told that they offend others when clothes are revealing. Women are told that masturbation is wrong or sinful, yet if a woman does not know how to please herself, she is considered frigid

> **She Should Know**
>
> Self-massage is a great technique for getting rid of any aches and pains she might have, but it can also be used as a part of sensual solo touching.

and unaware of what it takes to please a man. "Nice girls don't do that until they are married" has helped numb women to sexual pleasure and sexual feelings. For many women, it is an ongoing tug of war. Women have become so concerned about preserving their reputation that they fear experiencing any real sexual pleasure.

DEVELOPING HER SENSUAL RHYTHM

If ten women are asked to define the word *sensuality*, nine out of ten will say "sexy." In fact, sensuality is a unique dimension in and of itself, and not directly related to sex per se. Rather, to sense means to experience as it relates to all the senses—smell, taste, touch, sound, and sight. Since sex incorporates the use of the senses, raising a woman's level of sensual awareness and heightening sensitivity will play a major role in making her a responsive lover. When her sensuality is developed, she has found her rhythm.

Learning how to turn on means learning how to pay attention and tune in to her sexuality. The woman who is oblivious to her sexual feelings will be oblivious to her sexual needs. A sensuously tuned-in woman is responsive both inside and outside the bedroom. She has found her rhythm. She lives by the rhythm. Training to become more attentive takes considerable work, and discussing what feels good will help her find her own sexual rhythm.

To make her and her partner feel good, a woman can:

- Kiss him good-bye each day before leaving and upon returning.
- Make like spoons with him while sleeping. Get closer by touching, snuggling, and smooching.
- Spend the day running errands with him. Stop, have lunch, and run more errands. Plan dinner together and then head home for good lovemaking afterwards.
- Make sure they talk to one another each day about things that happened during the day. Take time to listen to one another.
- Say "thank you" when he does small things that he is supposed to do anyway. Help him feel appreciated.
- Compliment him. Tell him how good he looks and how good he smells.
- Touch, feel, and stroke his back. Compliment his body and his attitude on a daily basis.
- Reach for him and hold hands. Send messages of happiness to one another by touching for no reason at all. Encourage him to do the same.
- Snuggle every chance she gets.
- Practice simple acts of kindness.

- Clean, shop, dine, grocery shop together, and plan healthy activities with her children.

- Create sensual sparks that create passion by doing loving things together.

GETTING EXCITED

To get both her and her lover excited, a woman should do the following:

- Think of five things that bring a smile to her face every day.

- Keep a sexual journal that adds spark in the relationship when things get a little boring.

- Place love notes in numerous places throughout the home and car for her lover to read.

- Kiss for more than one minute several times every day.

- Plan romantic dates to rediscover passion.

- Enjoy a movie together.

- Wake him by giving loving kisses that create passion.

- Have moments of sensuous talk that encourage making love. Do this often.

TAKING HER FIRST STEP

Women have to pay attention to their physical and emotional needs. A woman can get away from the world's insanity and evolve by making her own music. Sex can become so good that it brings her ecstasy and makes her feel closer to her lover.

Good sex can make a woman throw up her hands, kick up her feet, and shout with joy. It can become so good to her that it brings her to tears. Women are eager to please their lovers and make them feel good. Sometimes they are so caught up in pleasing their lovers that they forget how important it is to find their own personal pleasure. A woman forgets that she really does like making love and sharing feelings of love and she forgets to incorporate what she likes. Before she begins to discover what feels good physically, she needs to take steps to get in touch with her emotional side. To find her way, here are some exercises she can do:

- Indulge in self-pleasuring. This exercise is designed to improve her memory skills. She begins by doing something very simple: going to a secluded spot, like the lounge or bed. She should bring assorted hard objects of many sizes and shapes, or have a close friend or lover bring the different objects to her secluded place. Examples are frozen links, cucumbers, carrots, bottles, soaps, and sponges—whatever makes her feel comfortable. She should close her eyes and let her body relax. Memorize and familiarize the feel of each object. Recall the size, shape, length, width, and texture. Think of each, and then contrast their differences. For a week, she should practice memory skills to increase her awareness of shapes, sizes, and textures. This improves her ability to touch in sensitive and caring ways. Another good thing for her to do is change out the items and discover how any new items come to life when touched with her eyes closed.

- Awaken her senses. In this exercise, she learns how to arouse her sexual appetite and awaken her senses. Practicing this exercise will allow her to move into this phase more easily. She should bring her mind, body, and favorite lotion. To help improve her senses, she can use the following exercises as a way to find mental pleasure in the smallest things. These exercises are designed to help the pleasure center of her brain. She imagines the wonderful pleasures by learning how to awaken the senses. She slowly moisturizes every part of the body while blindfolded and imagines the pleasure of it. With her eyes closed, she massages the scalp and shampoos. She might take a bath with her lover and wrestle naked playfully. She continues the fun after stepping out of the tub or shower by putting on some mellow music and dancing slowly to the beat of background music. She feels her body move and then controls the movements. She takes a shower in a darkened room with a small tea light candles and enjoy the sensuality and feel its presence. She reads *Keeping the Home Fires Burning* as erotically as possible. She makes sure she kisses him passionately every time he kisses her and gives full hugs every time she is embraced.

❦ Show appreciation. Showing appreciation makes her lover feel good about the relationship. Appreciation can take on many forms, from a phone call or compliment to a gift of flowers or a love note. She might dance for him while in the nude, wearing a pair of three-inch heels, or prepare his favorite meal while in the nude. But she should do something every day that her partner will appreciate. It takes only a small amount of effort and a little bit of creative imagination. Is that asking too much from her?

❦ Get away every now and again! Whether it is for a few hours, a day, or a weekend, she must create a little personal time. The best way to do this is by finding time to get away from everything and everybody. She should plan a special mini-retreat with her lover and be bold and creative. She should make this one of the most peaceful times planned. Then she might take her lover on a spicy romantic date. One way to change things up is to change her looks, her hair, and her setting, and do different activities. Making sure everything is positive and upbeat, she avoids arguing or bringing up any problems. This is a time of planned rejuvenation, escape, and coming together. It allows them to get lost in each other and shut out the outside world and its problems for a while. Sometimes it is nice to get lost.

❦ Have some fun. Romance and sex are fun! There is a reason it's called "foreplay." Duh! She and her lover should do something wild together. Visit an amusement park, arcade, or carnival without the kids! Play charades, strip poker, or Trivial Pursuit. Or go ballroom dancing or serenade each other under moonlight. A canoe ride can be very romantic. Romance is another word for "adult play." She should loosen up, be creative, and have the kind of fun and passion she had when she first started dating—and do it repeatedly!

❦ Fulfill fantasies. There is no reason to be embarrassed. We all have fantasies. She should do what turns him on and fulfills his desires. She might arrange that weekend away, or greet him at the door in a new (sexy) outfit—or in no outfit at all. She can rent a costume (be a nurse, police officer, firefighter, doctor, or whatever she desires). She should be creative in designing the evening around the best romantic fantasy ever.

❦ Turn ordinary into extraordinary. She can transform everyday events into mini-celebrations. Some fun suggestions include eating dinner by candlelight, enjoying breakfast or dinner in bed, taking a shower together using special soap, giving him a six-pack of his favorite beer for fixing the fence or doing the grocery shopping and then sharing.

❦ Be prepared for pleasure. She should always have on hand: champagne, candles, romantic music, massage oil, some of his favorite foods, great lingerie, small gifts, romantic cards, tickets to a special event, and take-out menus for when it's time to "get cooking."

- Cultivate a romantic psyche. Romance is not only a state of mind, it is an attitude. Romance is the art (not science) of expressing love. It starts by thinking as a couple first and second as individuals. It is how she does it that counts. Little heated gestures and sexy words are the glue that holds women together. Romance is not logical or predictable, so a woman should loosen up, get creative, and have some fun. Cultivating a romantic psyche will bring the heat back into the relationship.

- Take a break from the kids. She should do it for herself and her lover. She can pay the babysitter to take them out for the afternoon, or if all else fails, send them to bed early or place them in front of their favorite video with plenty of popcorn. Then she hangs a do not disturb sign on the bedroom door and pops her own corn.

When it is right, she will know it; and when it feels good,
she will want to do it again.

Chapter 11

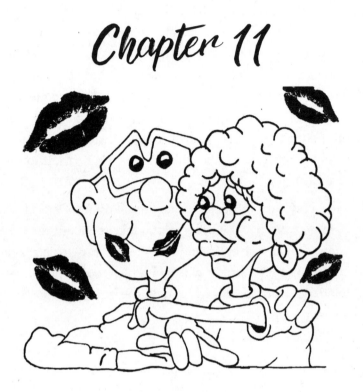

Her Sensuous Kisses

*Kissing is one of the most intimate acts of affection
a man and woman can share.*

Women love soul-searching kisses that pique passion, romantic interludes, and a desire to get lost in their partner. Was it the kind of kiss that
the woman did not want to end? Was it a deep, soul-searching kiss that
made her to want him badly, or was it the kiss that made her run to the
nearest bathroom and rinse her mouth out?

Many times the kiss is the first sign of true pleasure and sadly, men are unaware of this. Women really enjoy kissing, and if more men paid attention to the kiss, they could pass first base. Many women consider romantic kissing foreplay. A good kiss should be good, stimulating, pleasant, and fresh. A kiss should reach other parts of the woman's psyche: her brain, her senses, and most of all deep down in her soul.

Kissing is one of the most intimate acts of affection a man and woman can share. Yet, for most women it is the first act of affection and pleasure that is lost in a long-term relationship. If her sex life is missing stimulation, she can reinstate passion with kissing that will help her turn up the heat. To get the home fires burning here are some basics.

BREATHE: GET READY FOR KISSING

Bad breath will ruin a kiss faster than a woman can drop a dime. Bad breath occurs when the mouth becomes dry and stale, usually first thing in the morning or after eating certain foods. Alcohol, certain vegetables, smoking, and strong coffee may also make the breath stink. A woman should avoid foods such as cheese, garlic, onion, tuna, anchovies, salami, and sausages when kisses are on the schedule. These foods release odors for hours due to the oils in them. She should clean the breath before lip locking. To check her breath, she can discreetly lick the back of the hand, move it in front of the nose, and take a whiff. If her breath fails the sniff test, she should brush her teeth, tongue, and gums with toothpaste or mouthwash if possible. If brushing is impossible, she can drink some water, suck on a mint, or use breath freshener to make the kiss more appealing.

LIPS FOR KISSING

Lips have many nerve endings and are covered by a thin layer of skin. The softer and moister her lips, the more responsive they are to stimulation. Dry, rough, chapped lips are no fun for her partner to kiss and will provide less pleasure. To get the most from her lips, she should do the following:

- ❦ Wash lips daily with a clean, moist washcloth to clean and exfoliate.
- ❦ Apply lip balm during the winter months when lips tend to chap.
- ❦ Avoid licking the lips frequently, which dries them out.
- ❦ Remove lipstick before going to bed at night.
- ❦ Use long-lasting lipsticks in moderation, as they tend to dry lips also.

> **She Should Know**
>
> Depending on the culture and context, a kiss can express sentiments of love, passion, romance, sexual attraction, sexual activity, sexual arousal, affection, respect, greeting, friendship, peace, and good luck, among many others.

BECOMING A GOOD KISSER

The second step to becoming a good kisser is to keep the jaw and lips relaxed. Stiff, stingy lips make a man feel like he is kissing a vise. To prepare for great kissing, a woman should gather some breath mints or breath freshener and share with her partner. She can play some kissing games that will help her become more sensuous as she becomes better at kissing. To perfect her kissing skills, a woman should practice the following steps with her partner:

1. Part her lips slightly and brush them gently against his lips. Focus on the physical sensations as the nerve endings in her lips are stimulated.

2. Take his lower lip into her mouth as he takes her upper lip into his mouth; each should suck gently. Then switch. She can take his upper lip and offer him her lower one. Do this several times, each time getting better and better at doing it.

3. Smile at one another. Make this fun and sensuous practice time. Do not worry about technique too much; simply relax and go with the flow.

4. After a while, slowly open her lips a bit more, extend the tip of her tongue toward his mouth, and trace his lip from corner to corner.

5. Now begin relaxed mouth movements, using her tongue to sensuously play with his tongue. The initial contact with the tongue is quite arousing. Continue to touch and explore each other's tongue, moving both tongues up and down, side to side, in and out, and in circular motions. Sensuous kissing is like a sexy dance with the tongues—where couples play and chase, lead and follow, and dance back and forth with one another's playful ins and outs.

6. Keep playing and extend the tongue a little farther to explore his teeth, gums, and the roof of his mouth. Revel in the various textures, the stiffness of his lips, the slightly rough texture of his tongue, and the smoothness of his teeth. After a while, retreat and let him explore. Use her hands and fingers while kissing—rub his face, trace his mouth, massage his shoulders, rub his back, hold his face, run her fingers through his hair, wrap him in her arms and squeeze his butt.

7. Sensuously moan and groan while kissing to let him know how much she enjoys kissing him.

There is nothing worse than kissing a man who cannot kiss: his tongue barely enters her mouth, he barely touches her lips, and when he does, it darts in as fast as a snake and back out just as fast. Slow tongue action is more romantic and enticing. Face it: sometimes a woman will have to teach her partner how she likes to be kissed and vice versa. Playing this kissing game is a great learning experience for both parties.

HER EROTIC KISSING

Because his body is one huge pleasure zone filled with wonderful nerve endings, any part of the body will respond to licks, sucks, nips, gentle biting, and slight tugging. A woman should start by planting soft, gentle kisses on his forehead, cheeks, eyelids, earlobes, and neck, leaving his lips for last. This will make him eager to pull her mouth into his, but she should not let him—not yet. She wants to control these heated moments. She sensuously kisses down his chest, nipples, stomach, and navel areas. Still kissing him, she descends toward his pelvic area before detouring outward toward his hips. She slowly massages this area with a moistened tongue and then moves to his inner thighs, making sure not to touch his yearning penis area. This will tease him and set his soul on fire. He will try to direct a kiss to his penis, but she should resist it no matter how bad the desire is. Now, slowly move a little lower toward his knees and stay there a little while. This area gives him goosebumps, and he will squirm and wiggle with excitement. Then, she inches a little lower toward his shins and onward to the top of his feet and toward his toes. Kiss every part very slowly with lingering kisses at least twice. He will melt like butter.

Next, she reverses her direction and heads upward to his lips, taking her time to get there. She should kiss any part of the front of his body that was missed on the way down. She takes control of his body, slowly persuading him to roll over. While he is turning, she continues to kiss all the parts of his body: shoulders, back, spine, hips, buttocks, thighs, lower legs, calves, heels, and feet. She plants kisses everywhere and in the least likely places—she should get creative and surprise him. While covering his entire body with kisses, she lavishes his body with licks. Licking in and around the ear is a great turn-on for most men, just as long as she does not make loud, slurpy noises. Her motion is to lick down his spine, lingering on sensitive spots where his buttocks and spine meet. She licks across his skin, as if he were a lollipop, and notices his reaction. Next, she pulls his nipple into her mouth and kisses it around the areola.

It is very natural for women to move from kissing the mouth to other pleasurable parts of the body. The neck and throat are very sensitive areas to receive kissing, as are the breasts and nipples. It is pleasurable for both men and women to give and receive kisses, so a woman should try to do it often.

Women want to talk first, connect first, and then have sex.
For men, sex is the connection.
Sex is man's language of intimacy.

~Esther Perel

Chapter 12

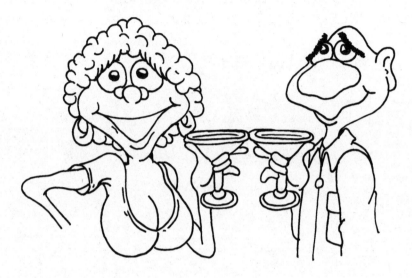

Celebrating Her Lover's Time

*To create a lover's night, she has to give him
some good old' fashioned pampering.*

A woman can get together with her partner for soothing, relaxing massages, beauty treatments, and good times by hosting a lover's night-in party. It is easy to turn a normal evening with him into a fantastic intimate party of pampering. Let's set the scene. It is about midnight on a Friday, and lavender aromatherapy scents fill the air. The evening is going great. Chilled wine, champagne, sparkling water, cold drinks, fresh vegetables, cheese, sliced fruit, and assorted meats are spread on a tray next to the bed. The sounds of soothing instrumental music fill the air. The environment feels good. With eyes closed and head cushioned, her feet are being massaged, all the while a smile is planted on her face. Maybe he is stretched out on a massage table too, lying in a semi-dark private room, enjoying a firm pair of hands working methodically over all parts of his stressed body.

She can choose to experience a soothing mudpack facial while wrapped in a fluffy white bathrobe, stretched out on a lounger with cucumbers on her eyes. The headphones are playing wonderful music while hot paraffin wax moisturizer soothes her hands and feet.

"This is simply divine." She feels so good she lets out a moan, saying, "God knows I needed this." Welcome to the latest embodiment of Lover's Time-In celebrations.

"It's a lot more intimate than a health spa," says Marva, a flight instructor. "And her time is not limited. It's very stimulating to get together with her partner to experience pampering, happy times, relationships, goals, and whatever."

She can share sexual fantasies with her lover, and what a great time to do it. Why not open up to her lover about some of her fantasies? Talking to each other during pampered moments naturally heals and educates. Sharing intimate secrets can enhance the pleasure. To create a lover's night, all she has to do is invite her lover over for some good ol' fashioned pampering, then work her magic on him. It is important that the environment is filled with trust, positive thoughts, and feelings in which all discussions are nonjudgmental and supportive.

FANTASY TIME

Both the woman and her lover should write down four or five sexual fantasies on index cards before meeting. When he arrives, his fantasies are placed in a large bowl with hers. After meeting and greeting, socializing, eating, and sipping on her favorite drink, it is time to read the fantasies. They each take turns pulling a fantasy from the bowl and reading it aloud to one another. She should get ready for laughs, rejuvenation, and shock. She will be surprised at how much she learns about

> ### She Should Know
>
> When talking about increasing sexual energy, we're talking about learning to leverage the types of energy she is already familiar with. For example, light, heat, sound vibrations, and her breath—along with intention—is the most powerful way to increase sexual energy.

sex just by listening to his fantasy. By the end of the fantasy, neither will be able hold back sensuous thoughts. Both will be anxious to get their hands on one another.

PASSION TIME

She should invite a local adult-store or Passion Party representative to give a presentation on erotic toys at her home. The sales associate will display erotic toys, explain how they work, and offer them for sale. This is a great learning experience. Passion Parties are to inform and educate women through tasteful in-home presentations. This is her opportunity to experience sensual products designed to enhance relationships.

FIELD TRIP TIME

Alternatively, she can plan a field trip with him to a local adult store to explore, sample, learn, and purchase. Both should take advantage of the wealth of knowledge available through the sales associates. They are eager to help people.

DINNER TIME

She can invite her lover over and have him write down his favorite recipes on several index cards. Place the cards in a bowl. When she is ready, she can take turns making dinner over several different dates. She can take turns selecting a different recipe to cook each week. She is responsible for selecting one or two of the recipes and making sure they are fulfilled within the next few weeks.

HER MASSAGE TIME

She should throw a sensual lover's massage party so they can both unwind, relax, and de-stress with the aid of a massage. Give him a range of complementary massages. Choose the types of massages that help couples relax and are accompanied by beauty treatments or other complementary therapies. Many spas bring every element of the massage with a custom menu of pampering. A woman can enjoy treatments in the comfort and convenience of her home with the same sensory details that she experience in a spa—aromatherapy, relaxing music, candles, robes, and slippers.

A sex symbol becomes a thing. I hate being a thing.

~Marilyn Monroe

Chapter 13

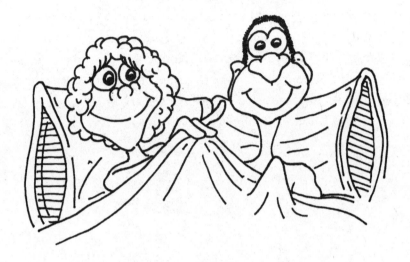

Bring On the Heat

A woman's bedroom should be her temple of comfort, relaxation, and pleasure.

Even little things such as the feel and texture of sheets can have a big effect on how inviting a woman's bedroom is. Because she will spend nearly one-third of her life asleep, the bedroom should be a place where she can go to renew at the beginning and relax at the end of each day. She should walk into her bedroom and run her hands across the bedspread and pillows. Are they soft and inviting? Are they warm and sensuous? Next she looks around the room. Is the atmosphere of her bedroom sensual? She can make her bed cozy by using cool cotton sheets during spring and autumn, crisp linen sheets in summer for a peaceful sleep, and cuddly flannel sheets and fluffy down comforters to create a cozy refuge in the wintertime. She may wish to lay plush carpeting or wear comfortable slippers to coddle her bare feet.

A woman's bedroom should be her temple of comfort, relaxation, and pleasure. It is not cluttered with

> **Body and Soul**
>
> Believe it or not, her genitals are not the most important part of the equation. What is of primary importance is the intention to build the sexual energy.

items that have nothing to do with sleep or pleasure. Her bed should have a sensuously yummy feel so that she can cuddle, make love, or drift peacefully to sleep.

To create this environment, she should remove any dirty piles of laundry and put away the exercise gear and the home computer. Bringing work and unnecessary items into the bedroom will cause her to associate the bedroom with negative emotions—stress, work, and clutter. This is negative anchoring.

By removing negative memories and associations from the bedroom, it will become a place where happiness is embraced and revitalized. A woman's bedroom is an expression of who she is. She should complement it with furnishings and beautiful items that reflect cleanliness, coziness, care, and concern. Everything placed in the bedroom whispers hints of her personality and what kind of woman she is.

Is the bedroom decorated in a way that nothing about her shows, or is personal flavor depicted in her surroundings? She should look around and see what her bedroom says about her. Is it cluttered, junky, dirty, messy, cold, drafty, insensitive, warm, inviting, conservative, imaginative, or sensitive? Is scenery important? Do others see her as a person who is caring, family oriented, faithful, neat, junky, messy, uncaring, religious, or romantic?

Is she cold or hot natured? Is she romantic or conventional? Is she a pack rat? Is she unclean? Does she feel healthy? Is she sensuous? Is she true to herself?

Starting today, she should set goals that will help the bedroom stay pure and true to her. As she considers what her bedroom says about her, she will become more tuned in to its presentation. She should replace the brightly lit lamps with flickering candles; the dirty linens with fresh, clean ones; and old, tattered, and torn rugs with rich carpet. New window treatments can replace old, outdated curtains or blinds.

> **Body and Soul**
>
> When she increases her sexual energy and starts to feel more and more turned on, she can use breath and sound to direct the sexual energy from her genitals throughout her body.

A collection of favorite scents should go where the computer once was. Sensuous or brightly colored magazines will brighten the room. Potpourri, flowers, and bright-colored candles help add beautiful touches here and there. Adding a few of his favorite things, or of his favorite colors, will make him feel welcome when he is in the room. If the relationship does not work, the decor can be changed to something else.

Over time, the bedroom will become associated with good times, good smells, good things, and sensuality. If the sensuous cues are powerful enough and the bedroom is free of negative anchors, she and her lover will experience an automatic and positive "sexy trance" upon entering her bedroom. Even if she lives in a small apartment or a home with limited space, she should not go crazy trying to make it the perfect room for pleasure. She should be practical and do the best possible. Once her sensuality plan is in place, she will begin to see and feel the quality. Her bedroom should denote sensuality more than sex. Now all she has to do is decide whether she wants to be sensuous or sexy, or both.

HER FIRST AND LAST IMPRESSIONS

To give the bedroom the sensual serenity of a private sanctuary, she should add details and treatments that are personal and chic. Bedrooms are meant for sleeping, reading, reflecting, romancing, pleasure, recharging, and escaping from the cares of the day.

Quality of sleep is very important for happiness, health, and productivity. To create the perfect bedroom, she should think about what she likes to do in the bedroom and define a style that is appropriate to her taste.

She must consider the bedroom as a sacred retreat. It

> **She Should Know**
>
> Said simply, sexual energy is her essential life force and a natural resource of the body that becomes highly charged by feelings of pleasure and arousal.

is very important that every object in the bedroom elicits a positive, nurturing response. She should strive for sensual instead of sexy. A cozy bedroom atmosphere invites rest and rejuvenation of the body, mind, and spirit. Comfort and safety felt in the world are connected to how safe and comfortable the home is—bedrooms included.

Here is the place to plunge into sensual fabrics, including chenille, flannel, silk, cotton, satin, or velvet. The view from her bed is very important: display a beautiful frame, a piece of art, or a vase of flowers that inspires her and makes her dream. The art in her bedroom makes a strong impact on her psyche, so why not make it a positive one? Sensual, serene, or romantic images will calm and inspire her. If she wants to honor her five senses, she focuses on creating truly sensual environments.

HER BEDROOM ENVIRONMENT

Before retiring at night, she should consider writing in a journal, reading, or reflecting on the day, rather than watching television. If she has a television in the bedroom, it should be stored in an armoire or cabinet when enjoying intimate moments with her partner. A pleasant bedroom environment can strengthen and nourish an intimate relationship. Placing importance on the bedroom environment can help her connect better with her lover.

Her bedroom should make a pleasing impression. The more active or hectic a woman's lifestyle, the more crucial it is that she have a private and appealing bedroom sanctuary in which she can rejuvenate and replenish pleasure. Women can nurture and enhance pleasure by thoughtfully creating a bedroom of allure, romance, and celebration.

> **She Should Know**
>
> Focus on diffused and layered lighting, as well as employing both shimmer and sensuous textures in order to create a sexy bedroom environment. The bold geometry with the contrast of soft diffused light creates a perfectly sexy bedroom.

HER BEDROOM STYLE

A woman can define the style of bedroom she wants. Comfort is the prevailing quality of all well-designed bedrooms. Clean lines are most relaxing, while others find plush opulence the most blissful. Bedrooms are as individual as the woman is. It is best to plan her bedroom design with private time in mind. She should add items that are engaging and delight the senses. If the bedroom is shared, ask her partner what he or she is relaxed by and then incorporate those ideas as well. Get struck with happiness each time the beautiful qualities of the bedroom come to mind. Consider several important factors.

A Relaxed Bedroom

Some of the most enjoyable ways to soothe the senses is paying attention to sight, hearing, smell, touch, and taste. A relaxed bedroom is the solution. She should imagine the most comforting bedroom she can think of: fluffy pillows, a lofty down comforter, a stream of natural light warming the room, soft colors and patterns, blond wood floors, and sheer draperies swaying in the breeze. The relaxed-style bedroom is made for sunny afternoon naps and leisurely weekend mornings spent reading in bed. It is soft, nurturing, and peaceful. It is perfect for a beachfront cottage or a cabin in the woods.

An Exotic Bedroom

If the exotic bedroom is her taste, all it takes are a venturesome spirit, a discerning eye, and imaginative details. The bedroom can become a temporary escape from the daily routine as it transports her to a tropical island. She should choose a statement piece: a unique bed, a distinctive piece of artwork or sculpture, or perhaps an exotic rug or fabric. She might opt for a plantation-style canopy and then stylize it with bamboo flooring, grass-cloth wall covering, and a large, breezy ceiling fan. Pairing materials in cool seaside hues with bleached drift-wood, or spicy Mediterranean colors with chiseled stone, will help set the right mood. Well-chosen accents, accessories, potted palms, tribal textiles, animal prints, and one-of-a-kind-lamps will reflect her sense of adventure. African drums create unique nightstands and accent tables. Asian temple doors make wonderful room separators or headboards. Beaded shawls and embroidered textiles fabricate fascinating pillows, draperies, and table runners. Tribal rugs make head-turning blankets. Incorporating these pieces into any decor instantly imparts the flavor of the land from which it came.

A Passion Boudoir

Today's homemakers plan for sex and decorate to create evocative, enticing bedrooms. A passion boudoir has flattering colors that contribute to personal beauty and are erotically appealing. Seductive colors, such as rouge and lipstick reds, creamy peaches, and subtle pinks, enhance natural beauty. A woman should be daring and use bold colors on the walls. Luscious fabrics will set the stage for sensuousness. Silky, velvety, and chenille textures can be combined with fluffy textures. A favorite decorator trick is to select fabrics that evoke a favorite-shared memory. Exotic patterns, such as animal or floral prints, create images of faraway journeys. Mirrors placed in unusual places, such as on top of dressers or on side tables, reflect dancing candlelight. Tropical plants and trees cast exciting shadows. The presence of a bed tray suggests the possibility of the ultimate pleasure: breakfast in bed. Soft lighting, candles, essential oils in a diffuser, and gentle oscillating fans effectively complete the decor in a passion boudoir.

A Bedroom Sanctuary

A woman can turn any bedroom into a personal retreat where she can escape and unwind from a busy day. A bedroom sanctuary surrounds her with photos of friends, family, and places she loves. Favorite artwork and meaningful mementos add to the atmosphere. Under-furnished private sanctuaries can also become a space to contemplate and daydream. Good colors for private sanctuaries include dark forest greens, deep chocolates, mochas, and navy or cobalt blues. Darker colors create a womb-like feeling and aid in deep sleep. A small refrigerator will help her enjoy time in the bedroom. Room-darkening window coverings encourage deep sleep and aid in the restoration of the soul.

A Bedroom Pleasure Zone

Here are a few simple things to make a bedroom into a pleasure zone that both she and her lover will enjoy. She can paint the walls a warm inviting color, purchase nightstands and lamps, and place a few erotic photos, books, and sensuous statuettes in strategic locations, along with several exotic plants. Use petals from a flower to tickle him from time to time. A fur rug or huge, soft, fluffy throw makes a nice addition to the bedroom. The fabrics used should invite touching, feeling, and comfort. Fabrics that feel like smooth silk, soft cotton, silky satin, rich velvet, overstuffed pillows, cozy comforters, and fluffy bedspreads are most inviting. These fabrics will make him want to touch her skin as well. Soft and sensuous music is essential in any bedroom pleasure zone, but she should compromise and play a few of his favorite tunes too. Once the music starts, she should find a reason to leave the room for a short while. This allows him to become relaxed while

She Should Know

Some of the most important elements of a sexy bedroom include soft sheets, dimmable lighting, candles, soft area rugs, and silk window panels. Another important feature is her mindset.

166

listening to his favorite music. Upon her return, she focuses on him and not the music. Pleasant scents can be scattered around the room. Fresh and clean are the best smells, but other scents will also enhance this pleasure zone.

ADD AMBIANCE TO ANY BEDROOM

Placing scents that he likes around the room will remind him of her when he smells those scents again. She should keep chilled wine or his favorite drink on hand. It is great for sipping before, during, and after intimate moments.

She wants to be sure to include his favorite finger foods and have plenty of fresh fruits and vegetables for him. The things he likes in bed should be a part of her "list of things to bring." And she must not forget the napkins. Soothing colored

> **She Should Know**
>
> She should be able to lower the lights to a dim glow when needed. Having multiple fixtures of different types allows mood change.

lights placed in various outlets will add a ton of ambiance. Red or pink lights are great! To help things get heated, they can dance sensuously while dimmed lights shadow the background.

Candles are great for soft lighting. Scented candles are even better. The flickering of the candlelight can help lovemaking become more exciting. She should make sure the bed linens are clean, fresh, and a pleasure to lie upon. Many pillows and soft, plush blankets are highly recommended.

A props and supplies box should be placed beside the bed (see Chapter 24, "Her Pleasure Containers"). The sex toys, games, condoms, body oils, scents, clean towels, tissues, erotic literature, and other sexual props are kept here. Battery-operated boyfriends (aka vibrators), silk scarves, beads, stockings, and breath mints, will help keep him in her in bed.

Find out what colors he likes and have touches of his favorite colors on hand. If he is crazy about jazz, she is sure to have jazz in her music collection. If he likes peanut butter, she has some for him. Whatever he likes, she is sure to have it. She should stock up, let the passion flow, and work on becoming the most sensuous woman he's ever met.

She should let him see her wearing the most sensuous clothing, so that when he leaves he'll still be thinking of her. An assortment of ribbed and studded condoms should be on hand. She might light a few candles and tell him he can do anything he likes—while they are lit.

A woman should live in the sexual moment, and keep her mind, body, and spirit where she is and with the person she is with.

A woman's bedroom should be her temple of comfort,
relaxation, and pleasure.

PART 4

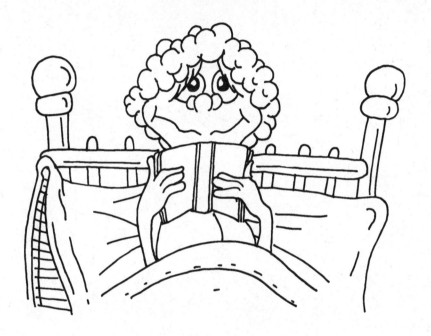

Stimulating Pleasures

Chapter 14

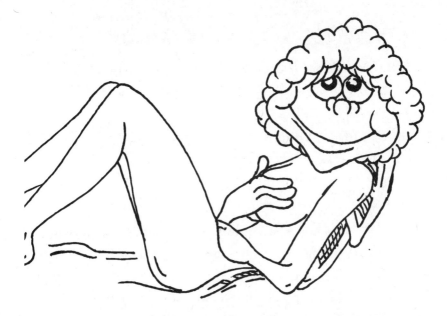

Self-Stimulating for the Woman

She can experience sensuality, touch, and pleasure with her lover.

When a woman really needs to get in the mood, the first and most important thing she should do is put herself in a sensual frame of mind. Every woman's level of sexuality varies in how she likes to get herself ready. Some women are able to get in the zone just by lying on the bed and reading an erotic story. Others may simply need to take a shower or a bath and rub on moisturizing cream under the flicker of a few candles. To get in the mood she can:

- Put on some relaxing background music to help ease into the mood.

- If sex toys are used, make sure they are nearby.

- Make sure she has privacy and will not be disturbed. Put the phone on silent and close the door. She will not want to be interrupted halfway to ecstasy.

- Now that she is in the mood, comfortable, relaxed, and feeling a little frisky, move to the next step.

FOR BEGINNERS

If she is a beginner at stimulation techniques, here is what she can do: lie on her back with her legs straight and bend her knees to expose more of her love button and vulva. Make sure the position feels comfortable, whether placing a vibrator directly on her love button or alongside it. When she is pleasuring herself, she does not have to feel pressure to have an orgasm; simply concentrate on what feels good.

Before a woman can experience sensuality, touch, and pleasure with her lover, it is important that she learn to explore her own body, to pleasure it, and to appreciate it. A woman cannot blame her lover for her failure to take off. She should take a good look at her sensual world, her relationship with herself, her sensuality, and her erotic sensibilities.

She Should Know

A sexually confident woman doesn't make men responsible for her pleasure and satisfaction. She understands and knows that her sexuality begins with her.

HER VIBRATORS

Once a woman has selected a vibrator, she should get to know it more intimately. Initially, she should experiment with her new toy when she's alone, so she can figure out what works best for her before she shares it with her partner. She should find a quiet, private place and carve out some "get to know her vibrator time." She should take her time and enjoy self-pleasuring without being disturbed. To increase pleasure and prevent friction burns, the use of some water-based lubricant to moisten the vagina and vulva, as well as the vibrator, will help. For the most pleasure, the lubricant should be kept at room temperature or a little warmer. If the vibrator is battery operated, she can warm the end of it in warm water. She can begin by asking herself a few questions:

1. "Have I experienced female self-pleasuring?"

2. "Am I aware of the sensual sensations of my body?"

3. "Am I aware of the feelings associated with my body, my sexuality, or my sexual power?"

4. "Do I know what words, actions, and touches give more pleasure?"

5. "Do I know what things relax my mind and body? Is it food, music, candles, or the feelings of silk on my skin?"

HER SELF-PLEASURING

Self-pleasure, or masturbation, is a great way to have some solo fun or just release a little tension. Masturbating relights her inner flame if her sex drive is somewhat lacking. Keep in mind that she is a powerful and beautiful sexual goddess and she deserves to be treated with respect, love, appreciation, and admiration. To do so, she should:

1. Set the mood. Create the scene. Prepare the ideal environ-ment, i.e., one that helps her relax and enhance her senses and sensuality.

2. Think music, lighting, fragrance, cushions, oils, toys, and clothing, or the lack of it.

3. Relax the mind, body, and soul. Have a slow, luxurious soak, or give him a massage.

4. Begin slowly by touching parts of her body (leaving the geni-tals until the end). Stroke, caress, and admire the body, hands, legs, and stomach. Admire the entire body. If any bad feelings come up, just note them and let them go.

5. Love on her. Continue touching and pleasuring, and make sure her last thoughts or feelings are positive, encouraging, and assuring.

6. Feel the positive and loving energy begin to flow around her body. She feels her skin start to tingle as the breathing deepens.

7. After at least twenty minutes of sensual self-touching, proceed to her intimate areas. Lightly caress the vagina, clitoris, lips, and any other area she wishes to explore!

8. If she experiences waves of intense pleasure and emotion, note them and breathe slowly and then deeply. Let these feelings flow. Always end on a positive thought and feeling. Continue with the female self-pleasuring.

9. Explore inner erotic beauty by inserting a finger slowly into the vagina—within an inch or two initially. Note the phys-ical and sensual sensations—the heat, moisture, and textures. Insert another finger if she is comfortable. Explore the vagina and G-spot, varying the touch. Drape a lovely silk scarf over

the area. Tease the clitoris, starting at the base of the clit and moving toward the head.

10. If she is indulging in intimate massage, making sure to use organic, cold-pressed, and virgin oils, such as almond, olive, and sesame. Do not use any essential oils in any form on or near the genitals.

11. Allow the powerful erotic and sensual sensations to build and flow in waves throughout the body. When she is close to climax, she should slow down, breathe deeply, and start again. Do this a number of times to allow a state of arousal for a good amount of time.

12. Enjoy the sensations until she cannot take it anymore. She claims and enjoys her female sexual power—the greatest power on the planet!

If touching feels good and the way she plans to go about it causes no risk of injury, then she should seriously go for it. Enjoy it. The more sex she has, the more her body wants and needs it. Masturbating two or three times a week can rapidly have her wanting more sex more often. Masturbation is a great way to for her find what turns her on, and what kinds of physical touching and fantasies will likely help her to reach orgasms.

STIMULATING HER BREASTS

Squeezing and flicking the nipples can add to the enjoyment of self-pleasuring. Her nipples will shrink and harden when aroused; sometimes just running a fingertip gently around the nipple can cause all kinds of wonderful sensations. There is no wrong or right way to masturbate, so she should not panic. She is dressed or undressed, sitting up or lying down—whatever feels good for her is the right way. She gets to know her body. Every nook and crevice could be holding some sensual delight, and if she does not explore, she will not find out.

STIMULATING HER VAGINA

Sometimes a woman wants nothing more than good penetrative sex. In this case, she needs to call in the trusty dildo. A dildo is a non-vibrating sex toy that will happily substitute for her man's penis. There are plenty on the market, and they come in an abundance of shapes and sizes.

With the dildo thrusting inside her, she still has a free hand to stimulate her clitoris. This gives her the best of both worlds. It takes a little more effort, but it is a lot of fun. She can always use her fingers if she does not like the idea of a dildo.

With great stimulation, the vagina lubricates. If a long time is spent here, even the juiciest vagina can start to dry out, so it never hurts to have a nice vaginal lubricant handy. K-Y Jelly can be found at any pharmacy, but there are many alternatives. But she should not use Vaseline or baby oil. Vaseline is too thick, and baby oil is too thin.

STIMULATING HER CLITORIS

Here is where more fun continues. Women are very lucky to have a clitoris. The purpose of the clitoris for a woman is to bring sexual pleasure. A woman should not underestimate the benefits of what role her clitoris plays in her sexuality. It is there for her pleasure and enjoyment only. When aroused, the clitoris grows a little bigger in size. It is the female version of the penis, so a woman can stroke it and play with it in much the same way. It is hers; she should not be afraid to play with it. She can begin by gently rubbing her fingers over the clitoris. For some women rubbing directly may be too much, so she can rub around the area of the clitoris for more indirect contact.

> **She Should Know**
>
> When a man wants to please her, she's not afraid to ask for what she wants and then be open to receiving it.

The more she experiments and gets to know how and where to touch herself, the better she will become at it. To discover the best feelings, she should play with it often. Her body will respond to her senses, and it will know exactly what feels good and what does not. When she begins to get excited, she can decide whether she wants to bring her vibrator or sex toy in on the fun.

A vibrator is great for more exciting stimulation. She can gently pass the head of the vibrator around the clitoral area, but she should not place it directly on the clitoris. Stimulating with the vibrator around the area of the clitoris, she can slowly move it toward, and then onto, the clit as she becomes more excited. If it is too sensitive, she can turn down the speed of the vibrations. A piece of fabric to put between her clitoris and the toy can also lessen the effect.

There are many vibrators to choose from, as with any toy. She can try different toys on different days with different speeds and vibrations. Using a lubricant when using sex toys is an option.

The removable showerhead is very sensually stimulating, using a setting that gives a steady stream of water, building up to a strong jet, and then moving it around so that the H_2O can stimulate the senses. She should be careful not to shoot strong streams of water into the vagina, as this could cause trapped air (which is not pleasant).

> **She Should Know**
>
> It's only through knowing her own body that she discovers what she wants and needs.

Some women like to rest with a pillow between their legs. She can try squeezing her thighs around the pillow or cushion, or any other soft object. Gently rocking the pelvis up and down causes the fabric to stimulate her clitoris. She is not touching herself, so it feels like someone else is. She should imagine rubbing against and squeezing on her man's thigh.

There are many ways to stimulate her pleasure spot. With all the above methods, it's best to start massaging the clitoris slowly and then building up intensity as it is touched and as she reaches her climax. As she climaxes, she should ease off, as it will be incredibly sensitive to touch. Sometimes, it is almost unbearable to touch the clitoris once orgasm is reached. On other occasions, she will be able to ride the orgasm into a second wave of ecstasy—these orgasms are the best.

STIMULATING HER G-SPOT

The infamous G-spot! The G-spot is the nickname for the Grafenberg spot, one of the most sensuous areas a woman possesses. It is analogous to the prostate in men, which seems to play a more direct role in sex and procreation. A woman's G-spot is a flat area about as big as a nickel, two inches inside the vagina. It is just behind the pubic bone, on the vagina wall that is closest to the belly button. She can reach it with her index finger. It is the gland located behind the pubic bone and around the urethra.

> **Giving and Receiving**
>
> She can use her hands or a vibrator to stimulate her clitoris as he hits her G-spot with each thrust.

If a woman is already aroused, stimulating this area leads to an intense orgasm of different quality than that of a love button orgasm. Stimulation of this spot produces a variety of initial feelings: tickle, slight discomfort, the need to urinate, or a unique yet pleasurable sensation. If the woman is not very aroused, she might have difficulty feeling it, and the man will have difficulty finding it. The trick is to get the genitals very aroused and then stimulate the G-spot. The best way to arouse is probably cunnilingus, which is Latin for having a lick, but any technique that provides good stimulation of the love button will do for starters. With additional fondling, this area may begin to swell, and the sensations may become more pleasurable.

Sustained stimulation may produce an intense orgasm. Like the prostate, the G-spot can produce a fluid like semen (but not as much), which may be released on orgasm—it is even known to "squirt" a couple of centimeters.

Plenty of foreplay is recommended before allowing a man to dive into the feminine area. At least half an hour or longer is fine. Once a state of interest is achieved, a woman can allow him to slowly start stimulating the love button (clitoris). Good love takes time. She should be careful, however, because the love

> **She Should Know**
>
> When in doubt, she should just come right out and ask what he likes during sex. Most men appreciate women who want to make sure they're satisfied. If he notices she's working hard to please him, he'll be more likely to return the favor.

button (clitoris) is very sensitive, and too much stimulation can cause irritation or chafing. In addition, different love buttons like different things. Some like very direct stimulation, and some prefer one side or the other, and others are so sensitive that they like fondling of the love button hood, or the labia. Some like a circular motion, and others like it flicked back and forth. The best way to find out what the love button likes is for a woman to pay attention to what feels good and what does not. She should start with some gentle experimenting. She must not get impatient; it can take a little while to figure out what works. Every woman's body is uniquely different.

A man can entertain himself by running his finger around the inside of the vagina, trying to learn more about its shape. If the female

> **Heated Moments**
>
> Even experts who have always believed in the G-spot weren't sure whether it was a gland or merely the collection of nerve endings extending from the underside of the clitoris.

is not coming (having an orgasm) or consciously causing contractions, the man will probably find that the vagina isn't doing anything in particular, just sitting there producing lubricant. If he brings his finger to the front wall of the vagina, he will find it less yielding than the rest, because there is a bone in front of it called the pubic bone, part of the pelvis. If he feels along this rigid section or just beyond it, he will find a slightly raised area. This is the G-spot. It might not be raised, but it will engorge once a woman becomes excited and starts to come.

He should not poke this spot or do anything with it because it will be distracting. He has to wait for the female to start to come. Now this might happen in thirty seconds, or it might take an hour. He has to be patient and keep his rhythm regular and smooth. Unless the female is coming, the man will find that the vagina is reasonably formfitting, although some are tighter or looser than others.

He'll be able to recognize she is coming when: 1) she tells him, 2) she moans a lot, 3) her breathing changes or escalates, 4) her face flushes, and 5) her neck, chest, and vagina begin to flutter rhythmically. A man may see and feel all these things or none of them. If he misses an orgasm, he should not stop unless he wants to, or she wants him to. Women have startling recuperative powers, particularly when they are receiving the right level of attention. Each lover should learn about one another's intimate need and desires. They should be willing to keep communication open by adding variety. Here are eight sensual favorites that women agreed they wanted and needed their lovers to do:

1. Rub the love button. The up-and-down motions usually work better than side-to-side or circular ones. Vary it from time to time, but up and down on the love button works best.

2. Push the finger in. When using a finger or two inside the vagina, one of the better motions is to push the finger all the way in, then bend it slightly when pulling it out, so that it slides against the top of the vagina. Not only does this feel great, but it also gives the man a chance at hitting her G-spot. If he does hit it, he will recognize he has done it by her reaction. He should work at finding her G-spot and use this knowledge to his advantage. Remember, that is the best place to rub when she is getting very close to orgasm.

3. Be consistent. A man can vary his fingering style, but he should not change it too often. When the woman is close to orgasm, he should not change unless she tells him to. He can move a little faster and pump his finger a little farther into her vagina, but he should not switch when she is near orgasm. It knocks her orgasm back a bit, and that can be frustrating.

4. Listen. Most importantly, when she is getting closer to orgasm, she will need the man to do something more. Harder, faster, rougher! She knows what she needs. It will help her orgasm if her man simply listens to her and does what she says. This is for her, after all.

5. Pay attention to more than the genital area. It takes a lot of concentration to get fingered. It makes her feel better and increases her general body sensitivity if he nips at her thighs, or rubs her stomach or breasts with his free hand. It helps her feel like she is more than genitals, and that means a lot to any woman's general pleasure. He might even stop from time to time to hug and kiss her. It gives both partners a break and preserves the pleasure.

6. Watch how she touches herself while he watches, and then he can pattern his motions after her. In fact, the first few times, he may want to ask her to finger herself so that he can watch. He should rub her love button, so that he can take care of one of those aspects. She can have him try more ways that make her feel good in other areas too.

7. Talk during the sex act. He can tell her she is pretty. He can ask if what he is doing feels good. She can tell him what she wants him to do and what she likes. That helps keep pleasure going, making her feel like more than a vagina.

8. He should not pull his finger out suddenly. Unless it is part of hard, fast thrusts, his finger should stay in or come out gradually. Ripping it out all at once is uncomfortable and painful. Sliding it very slowly can tease. He should make sure he looks in her eyes and smiles when he does this. She will love him more for it.

Communication helps both lovers find out what the other wants. If both lovers are willing and ready to learn, things will be just fine.

ONCE SHE STARTS TO RELEASE

Once the man believes that she is releasing, he should shift his attention from her love button to her G-spot. He should keep the same rhythm but use slightly more gentle pressure. He may want to keep some sort of contact with her love button, but just as his male identity (penis) becomes supersensitive during orgasm, to the point of discomfort, so can her love button.

> **Heated Moments**
>
> There's some disagreement about the size of the G-spot; it may range from a quarter of an inch to a couple of inches along the upper wall of the vagina—about an inch or two past the vaginal opening. Just as women are different so is the G-Spot.

As with the love button, he should pay attention to whether she pushes toward him or draws away from him, and he should try to gauge the amount of pressure he is giving. He probably will not need to vary his speed much, but he should pay attention to what she says she wants. She can help with this by telling him she likes the way it feels. If he is smart, he will catch on to her clues. If he is a little slow, she can help him do the things she likes.

As he goes for her G-spot, he will find that she will keep coming for longer than before. He may experience the sexual phenomenon of a female ejaculation. It is difficult to say whether the fluid comes from the vagina or the urethra. It is quite nice, sort of like ice cream. It is certainly not urine. The man should keep aiming for her G-spot. Eventually, he will feel her vagina draw away from his finger; it becomes fluffier, and the walls get taut and tight fitting, sort of like a little glove. When this happens, it is time to switch back to the love button moving with the same rhythm. When the vagina begins to contract, the lover should go back to the G-spot, keeping the rhythm smooth and continuous. The contractions mean she likes it and she wants more.

> **Body and Soul**
>
> The G-spot is its own entity, analogous to an organ in the male body. It's known as the female prostate because its tissue surrounds an area that produces chemicals similar to those made by the male gland that creates fluid to nourish sperm.

If he keeps this up for a while (and if her female genitals want to stop, then stop—this is not a competition), he will find that the nature of the vagina contractions changes. This does not mean she wants to stop; she simply needs a change of activity. The glove effect becomes less and less frequent, and he can spend more time with the G-spot. In addition, the contractions in her vagina become less simple squeezing and fluttering, and more a sort of reverse swallowing—a contraction that starts deep within the vagina and travels to its entrance. It feels like the vagina is trying to push his finger out.

Eventually he feels nothing but these push-out contractions, and he can go on as long as the woman wants to. (It takes time, patience, and many tries.) Hopefully his tongue and fingers do not wear out. If this goes on for a long time, he will need extra lubricant, which he should use if needed. Women have orgasms that last hours and seem to be much better than those that men can have.

A CLOSER LOOK AT HER STIMULATING PLEASURES

Except when aroused, the female genitals are usually detectable. The love button likes to hide under its own little hood; the lips stick pretty close to one another, and if the owner of the genitals is standing up and not aroused, she will not really see more than some enticing hair and maybe the outer lips.

Body and Soul

Some women say they experience a wetness unlike what they experience during other types of stimulation. Others say they even ejaculate a clear, odorless fluid upon orgasm that feels good.

A woman's genitals are more than "just a hole." Traditionally, all the sensations available from the female genitals derived from the lips and the love button, and it was thought that the interior of the vagina was practically numb to sexual sensation. However, that is not true because the vagina and its counterparts love to be touched.

A SENSUAL NOTE FOR HER

With the G-spot exercises, a woman will see increased vagina strength and control. When men practice penile exercises, which will be discussed in the next chapter, they will see increased ejaculation strength and sexual stamina. Both genders will see greatly increased pleasure and more intense, longer-lasting orgasms.

Sex never guarantees love, commitment, or even a phone call.

Chapter 15

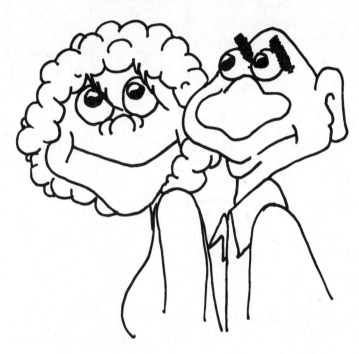

Stimulating Her Man

*For a woman, the male G-spot is not very difficult to find
and requires a little patience.*

First things first: every woman should look at and examine her man's
male identity (penis). I do not mean a short glance; it should not be
a hurried, surreptitious examination. She should also take time and
talk to him about it. She must convince him that some kind of treat

> **She Should Know**
>
> One sort of strange tip-off that she's found her G-spot is a sudden need to pee. Because it is so close to the urethra, touching it often triggers that feeling of having to urinate.

is in store for him, provided he will allow her to do pleasurable things with his male identity. The key is to make it fun and enjoy playing erotic games with him and his male identity. We have spent a considerable amount of time studying the female G-spot: how to find it, how to stimulate it, and how to turn a woman into putty with a G-spot orgasm. Men are far less familiar with is their own G-spot. The prostate is, essentially, the male equivalent of a woman's G-spot—but the woman's is far easier to find. Now it is time to find his in the most pleasant ways possible.

DISCOVERING HIS G-SPOT

In comparison, the prostate in men is also located behind the pubic bone and around the urethra. The two ejaculatory ducts also end here (bringing sperm from the testes via vas deferens). The prostate is reached through the anus (as in doctors performing a prostate exam). Continued massage-type stimulation of the prostate may produce intense orgasms in men. The prostate is the gland that produces most of the seminal fluid that is ejaculated (other than sperm in semen). The prostate can be considered the male G-spot. It is that sensitive.

Firm pressure is especially effective on the underside of the penis, where it is softer. Slow, firm pressure is effective and is certainly worth a try!

For a woman, the male G-spot is not very difficult to find but requires a little patience. The most comfortable position for this is while he is lying on his back, on either a bed or perhaps a large sofa. The process will be easiest with his legs elevated, which he can do by leaning his legs against the wall behind the bed or draping them over the back of the sofa. If a woman is having difficulty reaching his perineum from this position, she can lift his backside further by sliding a pillow or two under his butt.

Once he is comfortable, she should gently massage the area surrounding his anus. Most men enjoy having their perineum stimulated, and it can certainly be incorporated into the love session. Using her index finger, she gently explores. As he relaxes further, she can lube her finger and let it gently brush across the surface of his anus. Repeat this move several times, each time increasing the pressure slightly. If he is comfortable enough to let her probe, she keeps things slow and gentle, taking care to tell him to relax his sphincter during the process. Once she has encountered the male G-spot, she will recognize it as a small, chestnut-sized bump situated approximately two inches inward.

> **She Should Know**
>
> To help him find her G-spot, have him gently slip a finger or two inside of her vagina and then softly feel along her upper vaginal wall. If he is having trouble finding the right spot, encourage him to kiss or touch her nipples or outer V zone. The more aroused she is, the more her G-spot will stand out, making it easier to locate.

STIMULATING HIS G-SPOT

The first step in stimulating the male G-spot is making the man comfortable. Bathing beforehand can put a man at ease with the process, so start with a nice hot shower. If he would like to take that one-step further, enemas are not uncommon, and couples may choose to add this to their sensual regimen. Once he is ready for stimulation, there are a number of methods she can utilize. If the woman is a novice, a finger will be sufficient. There should be lubricant on hand, and it's best to get the type specifically created for anal play.

It will take some experimentation to discover what works best for him in terms of stimulation. They should return to one of the positions mentioned earlier (him on his back with his legs and backside elevated)

> **She Should Know**
>
> If she should find herself with a partner who is bigger than average, or even just bigger than what she's experienced before, when having sex, she should keep in mind that she should lubricate well first.

and repeat the steps used to locate the prostate. In preparation to stimulate his G-spot, she should keep in mind that some men enjoy gentle, thrusting movements, and some prefer intense, constant pressure on the prostate itself. He might prefer a mix of the two or something entirely different. She should give his body the chance to react and respond, taking time—his orgasm is worth it. It is also important to note that he may not find any of these methods pleasurable during the first exploration, and that is perfectly normal; they should simply try again in the future.

HIS MALE IDENTITY (PENIS)

Many women are concerned with penis size. Is it large or small or somewhere in between? No male body part has received greater attention than the size of his male identity. A man's obsession with the size of his male identity is probably a mental vestige of his primitive past, but as far as sexuality is concerned it's a waste of time.

A large penis does not have any effect on a woman's physical enjoyment unless she has a deep-seated psychological attachment to well-endowed men. Therefore, size only matters to the woman involved.

WHAT ABOUT THE MALE IDENTITY SHAPE (PENIS)

Is it curved like a boomerang or straight like an arrow? Is it short? Is it long? Is it wide or skinny? Does her fist fit around the spongy mass of the shaft? Does her hand completely engulf it? Can she squeeze it all at once?

Being able to appreciate his penis is good, but a woman should not be an organ grinder. She should be gentle yet firm. If the male identity has an unusual girth, her hand may not completely encircle it. In such cases, she can try both hands to ensure she does not miss any of his sensitive areas while stroking.

EXPLORING HIS MALE IDENTITY (PENIS)

A woman should explore every square inch of her man's genital area. She should look at his entire male identity—study it and learn its areas of special sensitivity and be ready to apply her knowledge to his body with her tongue and lips. To get from point A to point B, she should do the following:

- ❦ Look at it. Have him lie flat on his back in a well-lit room. Take his male identity

- ❦ (penis) and look at it. He probably will not have the willpower to remain soft. What man could stay soft when his lover is holding it, looking at it, and worshipping it?

- ❦ Touch it. When she is touching his male identity, it will become stiff and sensitive to stimulation by her lips, tongue, or hands. The first thing to note is the size of it, which should not make a difference at this point. Just hold it and respect it for a while. Once comfortable with holding it, move on to the next phase. Take time to notice whether he is circumcised, as she should know this about any penis she plays with.

- ❦ The shaft. Next, take a close look at the shaft of the male identity. There is a bulbous part of the organ near the outer end, slightly larger in diameter than the shaft that is called a "head." Technically, this is the glans of the male identity (this comes from the Latin glans, which means acorn). Look at it closely; it does kind of look like an acorn doesn't it?

- ❦ The outside. The outside perimeter of the glans is the corona. This joins the head to the shaft. This is the most sensitive spot on the male identity. It is toward this ridge that she will direct most of her attention when she is giving a blowjob. Follow this ridge around to the underside.

❦ Where is his most sensitive spot? Notice the point of juncture where the two ends of this irregular circle come together. If he is not circumcised, this is where the foreskin is attached. This tiny area is easily the most sensitive spot on his entire body, and it is possible to bring him to climax simply by gently tapping the tip of the tongue directly on it. Spend time caressing the glans and those areas immediately surrounding it.

❦ What is beneath the glans? Beneath the glans is the shaft. The shaft does not have many nerve endings and does not provide a high degree of stimulation for men either when caressed manually or with the tongue. Many women believe that sucking up and down on the shaft will get a man off. That is not necessarily true!

❦ The testicles. Beneath the shaft are the testicles (family jewels, or whatever she likes to call them, but let us not ignore their significance). The family jewels are extremely sensitive to pain, and a woman can add a high degree of pleasure for him by giving his family jewels the right kind of gentle attention.

❦ Where does semen spurt? Now let us go back to the shaft of the matter. The opening in the tip of the glans is the meatus. Here is where the semen spurts. She should roll her tongue around it, up and down on it, and spend valuable time here. It is very sensitive. Flicker and slap the tongue against it from time to time. He will love it. There is no greater love a woman can show for him than the attention she provides his male identity!

HIS CIRCUMCISED OR UNCIRCUMCISED MALE IDENTITY (PENIS)

Circumcision is not practiced by all cultures. During the Roman Empire, a man's foreskin (uncircumcised or draped) was important cosmetically to conform to the ideals of beauty. Athletic games required foreskin to cover the glans (head of the penis). Many athletes came from North Africa and the Eastern Mediterranean, where circumcision was common. Some physicians believed that circumcision was a means to discourage masturbation because it shortened the foreskin.

Circumcision became popular in the United States in the nineteenth century for the same

> **Watch Out**
>
> While many claim that circumcision is better for hygiene, it doesn't mean that a penis without foreskin can't smell. A smelly penis may have nothing to do with his penis. Pubic hair traps odors in the strands of hair themselves, as well as their accompanying oils. If it's not washed, it could lead to odor problems.

reason. Today, circumcision serves no purpose, and it certainly does not prevent masturbation, though it is suggested as a hygiene measure. A circumcised penis is easier to keep clean.

To clean an uncircumcised male identity (penis), a woman needs to spend a few seconds to get it clean. When erect, a circumcised and an uncircumcised penis look and feel about the same during sex. Some women refuse an uncircumcised lover's penis because of the extra skin. They feel that the uncircumcised male identity is not very attractive or is unclean. They feel that it is unhealthy to participate in sex with an uncircumcised male. This is a myth since most all men are born with an uncircumcised male identity.

TIMES HAVE CHANGED

When I wrote my first sexuality book, *Will the Real Women Please Stand Up* (Simon & Schuster, 1996), 62 percent of women I interviewed said that they would not dare perform oral sex on an uncircumcised male identity. Now, only 25 percent say they would not. I guess time really does bring about a change. From the first group, 46 percent felt that an uncircumcised male identity was unattractive and nonsexy, and that would keep them from making love to an uncircumcised man.

Today only 22 percent think an uncircumcised penis is unattractive, and do not feel that it would keep them from making love to a man. Of that same group, 15 percent felt that it carried an odor that was not very enticing when making love.

UNDERSTANDING PHIMOSIS OF THE MALE IDENTITY (PENIS)

There are men who experience the lack of a full erection due to the prepuce being too tight. This condition is phimosis. It is an abnormal constriction of the foreskin that prevents it from being drawn back to uncover the glans penis.

Phimosis is painful during urination and sexual intercourse because the foreskin does not willingly slide back and forth during handling. Sometimes medical circumcision is required when the foreskin is too tight due to phimosis causing recurring infections.

Circumcision on adult men is very painful and should not be performed purely for cosmetic reasons. Trying to circumcise oneself can result in mutilation and very serious infections.

REMEMBER THIS

As with any indulgence, there are advantages and disadvantages of sexual satisfaction. It can bring the highest kind of delight to a man or a woman. Try to understand both the pros and the cons of sexual indulgence.

Celebrate and honor her indulgence as well as her pleasures.

Chapter 16

Her Gratifying Hand Treats

Self-pleasuring is the first way a man learns to bring himself satisfaction.

Sex means more than intercourse. It means exploring all the variations that enhance a woman's sex life and keep it from getting stale. In deep, satisfying sex with her partner, it is a two-way street, and making her man feel good will also make her feel good.

Given that hand treats are fun and provide both partners pleasure, how in the world did it get to a point where women fail to recognize their benefits? For many centuries, masturbation was seen as something bad. Masturbation was forbidden because it could not lead to procreation. In the late 1770s, the belief was that masturbation, or self-touch of the genitals as some people refer to it, could cause disease of the body and even insanity, homosexuality, or hairy palms.

Of course, we now know better and understand that self-touch has many benefits. Women have reported that the orgasms they experience with self-touch are more intense. Women who experience masturbation as teenagers are more likely to be orgasmic during sex as adults. Self-touch has become one of the best ways for women to learn their bodies and become more aware of their personal pleasure cycle. Masturbation increases sexual self-esteem because women are not afraid to feel good about sex and sexuality.

Any woman can learn to make masturbation exciting. Masturbation is safe and normal, and feels very good. Mutual masturbation is a thrilling experience, but first there is a need to explore the basics of manual techniques.

Most men are afraid to let women handle their male identities. They feel that women are not skilled enough: their grips are too limp, they lack conviction or exuberance, and they are afraid to apply the correct amount of pressure. Further, some men believe that women pull or tug at inappropriate moments, disrupting the rhythm, or they scratch and do not pay attention to what they are doing. This means that women are in need of more information about the proper methods of hand masturbation.

HAND JOBS

Self-pleasuring is the first way a man learns to bring himself satisfaction. Maybe a hand job was the first thing a woman ever did with a man as she moved into her own sexual exploration. It might have happened early in her life, but this is no teenage thing. A hand job is an important part of adult fore-play. Women prefer to warm up to improved sexual experiences with the start of a hand job.

A woman will find that incor-porating hand techniques into her sexual experiences can bring about great sexual pleasure. This familiar and comfortable technique can bring a man to incredible and intense pleasure, especially if she takes the time to learn some variations on hand techniques. It can create some of the most pleasurable moments for him and her.

> ### She Should Know
>
> When it comes to sexual stim-ulation, men are not all the same. They have different likes and dislikes with regard to the kind of stimulation that works for them. Know a little more before you get moving.

GIVING HIM SOMETHING HE CAN FEEL

A woman does not want to pull, grab, yank, or squeeze madly on his crotch. Nor should she dig inside his pants and start tugging on his male identity as if he's a cow about to be being milked. That can hurt! Before she reaches for his male identity, she should take some time to relax him by warming him up with some gentle massaging. She should invest in massage oils that warm his genitals, or use reliable and odor-less massage oils. She can run it in her hands or place it in a nice dish that makes it easy to reach during a sensual massage. Massaging his male identity allows her to relax him before making love to him. The massage should start away from his genitals, maybe at his feet first or at his temples or his back. Step one is to place a generous amount of warmed oil in the palm of her hands and begin rubbing the muscles along the spine with long, slow strokes.

She starts by slowly sliding her hands all over his back. When she gets to his spine, she places her hands just above his buttocks, sliding them up toward his neck and shoulders and back down again. With each stroke, she widens the coverage so that she does not miss a spot. His body should receive equal attention from her smooth-flowing hands. Movements should be slow and rhythmic. Pressure should be slow and continuous.

> **Body and Soul**
>
> Romantic massages are more intimate and sensual than the average massage and can set the scene for a relaxed, couple-focused evening. Remember to take your time, focus on your partner, and enjoy connecting with them in new and exciting ways.

She varies the strokes, rubbing upward with one hand while the other travels down, making circles with both hands. She strokes outward and away from his spine and toward his waistline and back toward the spine again, taking care not to apply too much pressure. He should not feel like he is having a physical workout; he should feel relaxed and good.

She can make him feel better by using her oiled-down body to apply a sensuous massage to his body. By this, I mean she puts oil on her breasts, arms, and thighs, and uses them as tools to make him feel better. She uses her breasts to follow the same path as her hands. She uses her thighs to straddle his body while she is massaging him, sliding up and down his thighs while straddling him. Again, she uses her body to massage his body.

She also includes his arms and the backs of his legs, as well as his buttocks, an often-neglected pleasure zone. These large muscles hold a lot of tension; massaging this area can bring him a great degree of pleasure. She begins with nice, long strokes up and down the middle of the buttocks and then back up and down the sides. She varies the speed and direction of strokes by letting her fingers trickle up and down the palms of her hands. She takes the forefingers and strokes gently between his cheeks, making sure the scrotum is grazed with each passing. She does this several times until he is oohing and aaaahing.

Now, she asks him to reposition and assists him by gently helping him turn over, so his chest is massaged. Her strokes should be long, sensuous, sweeping motions similar to those used on his back. She can easily tease his nipples by slowing grazing over them with each massaging action. If he does not like her playing with his breasts, she can move just below them and massage his rib cage area. Sometimes he will like it here better.

Using the tips of the fore-fingers, she makes gentle and sensuous movement around his areola, being careful not to touch his breast if he does not like it. If he wants her to play with his breast, she makes tiny circles around it, every now and again applying little sucks with the front part of the lips. When his nipples are erect, she grazes over them again with a light touch of the palm of the hand. She continues this kind of massage until she is ready to move on, paying loving attention to his shoulders and his forearms, which are usually tight.

> **Heated Moments**
>
> A woman may be busy too, but she feels empty. Sensuality for her is not only a wave of pleasure in which she is bathed, but also a charge of electric joy at the contact with another. When a man lies in her womb, she is fulfilled, each act of love a taking of man within her, an act of birth and rebirth, of child rearing and man bearing.

Next, she moves to his legs, massaging his thighs, under his knees, above his knees, his calves, and his feet. When she reaches his inner thighs, she remains there for a while. She slides her oiled hands along his inner thigh, moving toward his sensitive areas and pausing just before she touches his genitals. Now, moving back toward his outer thigh and in toward his genitals, each stroke gets closer and closer to his scrotum until she is brushing it. If he is going crazy with excitement, she has done exactly what she was supposed to be doing.

POSITIONING FOR SEXUAL SUCCESS

The best position while giving a hand job is the one that is satisfying and comfortable for both partners. He should be relaxed and comfortable, and she should be able to move and massage his entire body with ease. She should be able to switch hand positions without straining to reach other parts of his body. She should be able to move with ease. It takes him a little longer to come while having a massage than it does while climaxing during sexual intercourse, but there are a few positions that can help her along the way. They are as follows:

- He lies on his back. She straddles his torso with her back to him, facing his penis.

- He lies on his back with his legs slightly apart. She kneels between his legs while facing him. This puts her in a position to use her thumbs to easily stroke his frenulum (the sensitive tissue on the back of the male identity where the shaft meets the head).

- He lies on his back. She kneels on either side of his torso or hips. She should not rest her elbows on his. It is painful.

- He stands. She sits on a bed, chair, or desk.

- She stands behind him and reaches around his body to his male identity.

- She kneels in front of him, placing a pillow under her knees for comfort.

- She lies on her back with her head on the pillows. He straddles her chest, balancing his weight on his knees.

- They both lie on their side facing one another, with her reaching down between his legs. He can stimulate her clitoris and while she plays with his male identity.

- She lies behind him. He lies on his side, allowing her to grasp his male identity.

BASIC STROKING

A woman can begin basic stroking by getting into her favorite position. A good position is where she kneels between his legs. Cupping well-lubricated hands over his genitals, she gets close to them but not quite touching. She gives him time to feel the warmth and flow of energy from her hands. Slowly lowering her hands until she is lightly touching him, covering his penis and scrotum, she lets her hands pause there for a few minutes before moving on.

With the slightly opened fist of her dominant hand, she wraps around the shaft of his penis with her thumb on the underside, along the ridge on the back, placing her thumb and index finger of her other hand at the base of the penis to stabilize it. She begins gently but firmly sliding up and down his shaft, sliding all the way down to the base of his penis. As she slides up toward his male identity head,

> **Heated Moments**
>
> The manner in which a woman and a man connects sensuously adds to their sexual appeal. Its like a romantic bowl of beautiful flowers twisting, turning and finally joining as one fulfilling delight.

she uses a tighter grip. Then she slides all the way down toward the bottom of his male identity and continues with smooth, steady rhythm—up, down, up, down. She begins slowly and increases speed, and as he begins to get harder, he will give her physical signs that he wants more.

ACHIEVING MORE FROM HER HAND JOBS

As a woman gets more comfortable with the basic strokes, she might explore some of the following techniques.

- Begin with the basic stroke. When her hand reaches the head of the male identity, she twists the palm of the hand completely over the head of the penis as if rubbing it and then continues with the downward stroke.

- Begin with the basic stroke. She lubricates the thumb, and as she slowly slides her hand up and down his penis, moves her thumb quickly, up and down in nice circles against the underside of his frenulum.

- Begin with the basic stroke. When her hand reaches the male identity head, she twists her hand in one direction and continues down to the base of the penis.

- With her thumb and index finger, she makes the shape of the letter *O*. Slide the *O* over the head of the penis and move it up and down the shaft. After a while, she lengthens the stroke, tightens the grip nearing the corona of the head, and slides the fingers up and over the head and then back down again.

- Starting with the letter *O* movement as stated above but sliding the index finger and thumb up to the head, she twists her fingers at the base of the penis to stabilize it. She lubricates the palm of the dominant hand and slides it up and down the back of the penis. To add interest, she slides one hand down his scrotum to his perineum while the other hand slides up along his penis. In this one, her hands will move away from one another.

- She wraps her hands around his male identity, with her thumb at the base of his penis and her baby finger resting against the head. Her hand will be upside down, and she should slide her hand up and down. This technique works well if she kneels at his side.

- While cupping his male identity in the palm of her hands, with her fingers pointing down toward his scrotum, she grips the sides of his penis and rotates the palm of her hands in one direction and then the other.

TECHNIQUES FOR USING BOTH HANDS

To heighten the excitement, a woman can do the following:

1. Place both well-lubricated fists around his penis, one on top of the other. Move the hands in unison up and down the entire length of his penis. He will get a sensation similar to thrusting into a tight vagina.

2. Place both hands as above, but move them up and down and, twist both hands together in one direction and then in the other. Add more interest by twisting one hand in one direction and the other hand in the opposite direction.

3. Lace the fingers of both hands together and encircle his penis. The thumbs should be free, positioned at the level of the frenulum. Now, keeping the hands still, move just the thumbs up and down in opposite directions along the frenulum, varying the speed and pressure.

4. Interlock the hands as above but lace them together this time. Slide the interlocked hands up and down his male identity.

5. Grasp his male identity head with the right hand and slide it down to the base. When she reaches the base, she will place her left hand on the head and slide it down. Releasing her right hand, she returns to the head. Repeat with alternating hands.

6. Grasp the head of his male identity with the right hand and use the same alternating technique as above, except slide only the right hand down to just below the head before starting with the left. Alternate hands for several rapid strokes. This works best with an erect male identity.

7. This is the opposite of the one above. Place the right hand around the base of his penis and slide it up and over the head. As she reaches the head, begin the same upward movement with the left hand. Repeat with alternating hands.

8. Begin just below the head and slide up over the head and back down to an inch or two below it. Repeat for several rapid strokes before returning to the longer strokes described above. This technique may be used on a flaccid penis, but do not expect it to remain in this state for long.

9. Form the *O* sign with the thumb and index finger of each hand. Place both the *O*'s around his penis. Now slide one hand up and just over the corona, while moving the other down to the base of the penis. Move both *O*'s back and forth. Add more intensity by twisting the hands as they move up and down.

10. Place the palm of the hands on both sides of the penis. Gently rub the hands back and forth, in opposite directions, along the side of the penis as if starting a fire.

ENHANCING HER HAND JOBS

1. The best way to please a man with hand jobs is to watch what he does while pleasing himself. She should ask him to help with learning the moves he likes, or be a little bolder and ask him to show by demonstrating his favorite moves. If he is shy about showing her how, she should ask him to place her hand on his male identity the way he likes it. Then have him place his hand on top of hers and move it the way he likes it on his male identity. He can show her how much pressure he likes and what speeds are best.

2. She shows him that she likes what he is doing. He needs to know that she is excited about giving him pleasure.

3. She should honor his penis. She should tell him how much she likes his penis, how much she likes playing with it, and how much she likes holding on to it.

4. She should focus all attention on him and provide unselfish gestures of love by giving him stimulation, while taking her time.

5. She must communicate effectively. She asks questions about her pleasures and his. It is essential to understand what he likes, wants, and needs by communicating that she wants to please him.

6. She begins with nice, even, continuous strokes.

7. She has a great lubricant available for hand jobs.

8. She stimulates by using both hands when massaging him.

9. She should alternate and vary hand job movements, switching from one technique to the other with grace and rhythm.

10. She continues gentle stimulation and watches him for hints of "I want more."

UPGRADING HER HAND TECHNIQUES

Once she gets comfortable with the basic and advanced hand moves, she moves on to techniques that are more complicated. To perfect her advanced hand skills, a woman should:

1. Avoid stroking or jerking on his male identity. Feel the fullness of it by letting her fingers smoothly run from the family jewels to the top of his male identity.

2. When giving him a hand job, swirl around and then slide back down to the other half, back down at his family jewels. The

movements should be steady and smooth, without bumping, stalling, or nicking him.

3. Tease the more sensitive areas of his male identity. These include the glans and corona, and the tender parts of the bottom side of his male identity, where the long vein is located. Look at it.

4. Bring the palm of her hands up to the top of the glans and place it flat out with the fingers held together and stiff, thumbs pointed straight out. Spin it around as if removing the lid of a jar. He will moan and groan with delight. Because his glans is supersensitive, this motion will bring him to high levels of pleasure. While she is performing this skill, he might try to push her hand away, but he will love it. Even though he will plead a break, he does not mean really it. It will drive him crazy with pleasure.

5. Slip the hands down to his jewels and ever so gently, so she can hold them in her fingers, softly tug them down away from his shaft. If they are big and bulky, like grade AA eggs, bounce them up and down a couple of times in the hands. Tell him how heavy they feel and how sexy they are. Caress them gently but never, ever squeeze them.

6. Notice that one of his family jewels hangs lower than the other. This is perfectly normal. Once she feels comfortable with the way his family jewels feel in her hands, gently roll them up the underside of his shaft. Depending on their size and the amount of room in the scrotum, they might reach halfway down his penis. He will like the way this feels. It is pleasurable to him.

7. After letting go of his jewels, bring the fingers together in a makeshift goose head formation. Very lightly begin to stroke his erection with the fingers, running them all over his sensitive

shaft and family jewels. She may wish to slip the pocket of her goose head handhold over the tip of his male identity, letting it rest there for a few seconds. This really excites him.

8. About this time, his male identity will probably start to emit its natural lubricant. Pre-seminal fluid is nature's way of moistening the canal of the urethra so that the spermatozoa can swim more easily out of it; it also lubricates the head of the male identity. An uncircumcised male identity gathers up this lubricant within the foreskin and keeps the head very moist and slick. Use the juice to lubricate the shaft. It has a musky smell, which is an aromatic aphrodisiac during pre-love sessions.

9. Add a drop of moisturizing lotion to the shaft and gently rub it in. Massage the lotion between the hands before putting it on the male identity because sometimes the cream is cold. Rubbing warms it.

10. Invest in a warming lotion. If he does not seem to have a very firm erection, try using a cinnamon-based ointment, which can be found at a local sex novelty store or acquired through a mail order catalog. The slight warming sensation often causes the male identity to become rock hard.

HAND JOB EXERCISES

The following exercises were written with an experienced woman in mind. But any woman can try any of the techniques that interest her, or him.

❦ Switch hitter. Using both hands, she alternates back and forth in a pattern to offer him the most arousal. He will notice the difference. She should not get into a routine where the strokes are dull and noncommittal. By giving it to him good, she gets him to the point where he is singing with happiness.

❦ Double whammy. Some male identities are so big they require both hands. A woman can use one of her hands to caress and lightly flutter his family jewels, or tighten around the base of his shaft. If both hands fit along the length of the shaft, she moves them together, up and down, in the typical pumping motion. She should imagine herself holding a baseball bat and about to score a grand slam. She varies the directions of her hands, one up, one down at the same time. Two hands are better than one.

❦ The anvil stroke. She brings one hand down, letting it stroke the male identity from the top to the bottom. When it hits the bottom, she releases it. Meanwhile, she brings the corresponding hand down to the top of the shaft, creating an alternating beating motion—hence the name "anvil stroke." Think of those blacksmith duos that keep up a double-beat pounding motion as they beat that rod of iron on a piping-hot anvil.

❦ The shuttle. Not many people have heard of the "shuttle," but it is one of the best. She takes the male identity in both hands, fingers lightly touching the sides of the shaft. In order to visualize the position, she should think of holding a clarinet. Now she flicks the male identity back and forth between both hands by holding on to the loose skin of the shaft. Shuttling it back and forth in this manner may not seem incredibly thrilling to him at first, but soon, as it builds up momentum, it will drive him out of his mind.

❦ The bookends. She places both hands side by side against his shaft like a pair of bookends. Now she pushes hard against his male identity and lifts both hands up and down. She continues in this manner for a while. The constant tugging of the skin around the family jewels and the mons pubis will do the trick.

❦ The flame. She places both hands gently on either side with fingers pointing away from the male identity. Then she rolls his male identity between both hands like a stick of wood to keep the home fires burning for a long time to come.

❦ The base clutch. She tightens the thumb and forefinger around the base of the shaft, pressing down on the family jewels. This will cut off the blood (acting as an impromptu male identity ring) and help steady the shaft in the hand. If the skin on it is slick and immutable, she strokes the male identity with more friction, thereby enhancing the excruciating experience.

❦ The love tug. While stroking him, she lovingly pulls on the wispy strands of pubic hair sprouting from his testicles. Not pulling too hard or fast, she teases them gently.

❦ The two-timer. One of her hands tickles his family jewels while the other massages him upward then downward.

❦ The thigh swatter. She uses the hand that is currently unemployed to firmly but lovingly stroke his inner thighs.

❦ The best fist forward. She places one fist against his perineum (the skin between the butthole and the balls) while stroking him. He will probably start opening his legs a little wider, giving more space to press against his perineum. This is one is guaranteed to drive him wild.

❦ Making buttermilk. She places the palms of the hands on both sides of his penis and rubs the hands in opposite directions up and down the full length of his penis—as one goes up, the other goes down.

❦ Touch and go. He gets in doggy-style position on both his hands and knees as she kneels behind him and reaches between his legs. She strokes his scrotum, wraps the other hand around his penis, and begins basic up and down strokes. As he becomes aroused, she plants kisses on his buttocks and, if she can reach them, his anus and his scrotum. It will drive him wild.

🐝 Head to head. In his favorite position that allows her to face him, she begins with the basic stroke. As he becomes aroused, she places her mouth over the head of his male identity with the lips fitting snuggly in the groove beneath the corona. She continues to stroke with the hand, while flicking the tip of the head with the tongue.

🐝 The sleeve. He lies on his back as she begins the basic stroke or one of the variations. While stroking with one hand, she reaches for a well-lubricated penis sleeve with the other (see Chapter 24, "Her Sex Toys, Lovers' Props, and Supplies"). She slides the sleeve over his erect penis and moves it up and down, using the basic stroke. The sleeve gives him a sensation much like the vagina; he will love it.

🐝 Going marbles. She places several small marbles in a glass of water. He lies on his back, and she begins the basic stroke. As he becomes aroused, she slips a small marble into her palm and gently strokes his penis. The marble will move smoothly along his penis, adding layers of sensations. As he becomes more comfortable, she adds one or two more marbles, keeping the grip light to allow the marbles to move. She does not grip too hard.

🐝 The seesaw. She places a latex plastic glove on her dominant hand, lubricates it well, and then, holding his penis in her hand, begins the basic up and down or any of the variations.

🐝 Water soak. She runs a warm bath for him, adding moisturizing bath oil or baby oil to the water. As he soaks, she kneels at the side of the tub, reaching into the water, and begins to massage and stroke his penis. The warm water will increase his blood flow, and the water will act as a nice, steady lubricant, making the hand movements easier. She can change the sensations a bit by lubricating her hands with a long-lasting, water-based lubricant that is stable underwater. The lubricant Eros Body Glide is great for underwater play, which will be discussed later. If she wants more excitement, she can slip into the water and let her nipples and water-soaked body glide against him.

❦ Good vibrations. She slides a finger vibrator onto the middle finger. While stroking his penis, she cups the other hand gently over his scrotum and presses the vibrating finger against his perineum. The vibrations will spread to his G-spot and drive him wild.

❦ Vibrator slide. She places a hand vibrator over the back of the hand, lubricates her palm, and slides the hand up and down the shaft of his penis. With every two or three up strokes, she slides the hands over the head of his penis and then back down his shaft.

❦ The barrel. He stands while she sits on the bed or a chair. Lubricating both of her hands well with warm oil or silicone-based lubricant, she forms a barrel by making two open fists and placing one hand on top of the other. She slides the barrel over his penis and remains still. To add variety, she can squeeze his penis tight as he pulls back and loosen the hands as he thrusts forward. Squeeze and release the fingers rhythmically to create sensations similar to those she creates when she squeezes his pubococcygeus (PC) muscle, located in the perineum area behind the scrotum and in front of the anus. PC muscle exercises improve the sexual performance in men by delaying ejaculation at will.

To become the best at pleasing him, I recommend that a woman study her own wants, needs, and desires, and then incorporate what

> **Body and Soul**
>
> A huge benefit of a hand job is that it can be done sneakily. If she wanted to get a hand job going while sitting side-by-side on the couch while watching a movie, that would be good and acceptable.

she likes into her own sexual relationship. She should explore the outer limits of sensuality—get out of the routine of doing what she has always done and then do something that she has never done before.

She's a woman who prefers additional stimulation—a finger or two inside the vagina, or perhaps even the anus. Some want the man's hands to reach up and play with her breasts, or want his fingers to hold her labia apart so that his tongue can get at her vulva more directly.

As a woman nears climax, she prefers stimulation that is more direct. In general, fast, rhythmic stimulation is most effective at causing climax, but the man should not rush to get there. He should always take his time and learn what he can do. Most men who enjoy cunnilingus agree that a clean vagina is a pleasantly acquired taste, so woman should wash first to be rid of any bothersome, unwanted, or unnecessary odors.

Get excited about trying new things that will improve pleasure.

Chapter 17

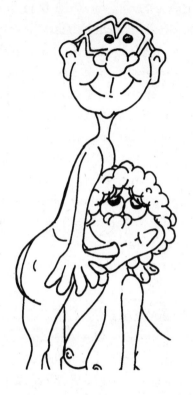

Her Gratifying Oral Sex Treats

Getting good oral sex is like receiving a precious gift.

Performing oral sex takes some courage (at least the first time). At lot of people are afraid they will find the smell and the taste repulsive. A woman may never like the taste of semen, but over time, she gets used to it, as does a man who indulges in oral sex with a woman. A woman's sex organs usually taste and smell more intensely than a man's smell. That is because of their tight, compact, and enclosed structure.

If the smell of the woman bothers the man, he can use something to cover the taste and smell, like chocolate, a favorite sauce, or jam. He should be sure to use something that does not cause rash or irritations and take care not to get any of these flavors inside the vagina. A dab here or there on the inner thighs is quite nice. He can go back and forth, tasting it from time to time at different intervals.

If the smell of the man is not enjoyable to the woman, she can take a shower with him and participate in cleaning him. That is also fun. They should be sure to clean the teeth, gums, and breath before oral sex, and remember the mouth has more germs than a clean male identity or vagina. I hope that this information will help first-timers break down any barriers, which might prevent them from expressing their love and receiving great oral fun from a companion.

THE PLEASURE OF CUNNILINGUS

Getting good cunnilingus is like receiving a precious gift. When performed well, it provides women with intense pleasure. In fact, it is the easiest way for women to experience an orgasm. If the man is a little apprehensive about trying cunnilingus, it is important for the woman to let him know how much she would like to experience this form of oral pleasure. She can help him get rid of any fears he might have about hygiene (a common male concern) by offering to shower together prior to sex. If it's lack of experience that causes him concern, she can agree to work with him to help him develop his own unique cunnilingus style. She can offer him one of my books or choose one of many sex guides that are devoted to the art of cunnilingus and then they can read it together.

There is no excuse for a man to refuse to provide her with oral pleasure. To fully enjoy the pleasure of cunnilingus, a woman should:

1. Check her genital attitude. How does she feel about the appearance, smell, and taste of her own genitals? She is not alone if her answer is "not good." Some women are not comfortable with their most intimate parts. She has probably been conditioned since childhood to think of her genitals as unattractive, smelly, or unclean. Having him get up close and personal to her genitals can make her feel slightly uncomfortable. She might think that he also finds the feminine anatomy unattractive, and she might think he is turned off by her taste and smell. She should not feel this way because most men find a woman's genitals very attractive and sexually enticing.

2. Get in tune with her own genitals. Take a closer look at them with a handheld mirror. Appreciate the genitals' color, texture, moisture, and complexity. Become familiar with their unique scent. Place a clean finger in the vagina. Remove it, wave it several inches from the nose, and breathe in its scent. Take a deep breath and enjoy how it smells. The natural, clean-smelling vagina is very powerful and erotic to men. Now take the same finger, place it in the mouth, and taste the secretions. The flavor of the vaginal fluids may range from sweet to slightly salty to no taste at all. The taste may vary throughout the month and be affected by whatever has been eaten, drunk, or smoked. Cigarettes, alcohol, recreational drugs, medications, vitamins, coffee, and such foods as onions, asparagus, garlic, and curry may give the genitals a less-than-pleasant taste. Eating lots of fresh fruits and vegetables and drinking lots of water will help keep the unique vaginal taste favorable and fresh, giving it a sweet taste.

3. Learn to receive pleasure. Because so many women are givers, sometimes it is the most difficult thing in the world for a woman to receive pleasure. In order to reach the heights of sexual pleasure, she must be able to concentrate on her own

pleasure. Cunnilingus is the perfect opportunity to lie back, forget her worries, and get pleasured by her mate.

- ❦ His pleasure is dependent on her pleasure. Few things will make her partner happier than being able to give her the ultimate sexual experience. Men are like that. They want to think that they are the reason for her happiness and pleasure.

- ❦ Orgasms should not be the ultimate goal at this point, so please do not worry about how long it will take to get one. Relax and concentrate on the pleasure received.

4. Choose a good position. She should find a comfortable position that is good for her. She needs to be relaxed in order to feel good sensations. The best position is when she lies on her back with her knees bent and he lies between her legs. This position gives his tongue and mouth the best access to the sensitive part of her clitoris and vagina. Propping her butt on pillows increases access to her vagina and buttocks.

5. Make sure he is comfortable. Be sure to have plenty of pillows available to support his joints and other body parts. Make sure that she moves far up enough on the bed or table so that he has enough room to get into a comfortable position.

- ❦ Place fresh water at the bedside just in case he needs to replenish his saliva. Flavored lubricants and gels may add variety and spice to his lovemaking, but may irritate the genitals. Be sure to select no allergenic gels, creams, and so forth.

6. Communicate her needs. As with any sexual activity, communication is the key. Do not expect him to know what she wants or need. Men assume that the penis and the clitoris want and need the same treatment. When it comes to oral pleasuring,

nothing is further from the truth. The average penis and love button like to be fondled, kissed, and sucked. Use her body language to give him feedback and direction on how to provide pleasure to her. Move and glide the pelvis to direct his tongue to meet the sensitive spots. Move side to side, thrusting the pelvis closer to get more attention and farther away if the stimulation is too intense.

🐏 For additional stimulation of the G-spot, perineum, or anus, gently guide his hands to that spot. He will then know what she wants and needs to be pleasured.

7. Vocalize pleasure. When she is silent, he might think that she is not interested or bored with his lovemaking. He might think that he is not doing a good enough job. If she displays this kind of attitude, he will lose interest in making love to her. She has to moan, groan, coo, oooh, and aaaah with pleasure to let him know that it feels good to her. Express pleasure and he will want to do it repeatedly.

8. Give him a hand. Become more of an active participant than a passive participant. He needs to know that she wants him just as much as she needs to know he wants her. Get involved by pulling her love button hood back. Play with the vagina, nipples, or other erogenous zones that increase arousal.

9. Stroke the back of his head, rub his buttocks, run fingers through his hair, massage his arms, talk to him, and let him know it is all good. Kiss him immediately afterwards. Show him that she is comfortable with her juices by kissing him and tasting her own love juices.

10. Show appreciation. Let him know how much the cunnilingus is enjoyed. Most men love to pleasure women. Knowing that

he pleased her will make it more likely that he will be eager to do it repeatedly. Remember, the pursuit of pleasure requires relaxation.

CUNNILINGUS DURING MENSTRUATION

Some people are grossed out at the suggestion of cunnilingus during menstruation. If it is a concern to a man, the woman should wait. A tampon may well hold the flood back, as will a diaphragm, but some men do not like the taste of a menstruating vagina. If both partners are healthy, however, there is no particular danger in menstrual blood, and some women find that orgasms during their periods alleviate cramps. It is purely a matter of personal preference.

FELLATIO

Fellatio is giving a blowjob or sucking a man's male identity. It is the act of applying lips to a man with the purpose of giving him pleasure. It is one of the pure male pleasures in life. Many women do not appreciate just how much fun it is because they do not know how to do it correctly or they have a phobia about it. When it is done wrong, the male identity does not get hard, the man does not have a good time, and the woman feels like a sexual failure. The lips and the tongue are the major sources of stimulation for what makes it feel good to the man. Both men and women respond well to direct pressure and continuous rhythm, so a steady, strong stroke will be enough to give the proper stimulation.

> **She Should Know**
>
> First, she should stop thinking of oral sex as a job. Done correctly, oral sex can be satisfying for both partners.

The best way to give fellatio is still with the lips and tongue, taking only as much as she can without gagging. However, if a couple wants to take it further, all they have to do is practice. It is simple: she takes his male identity without choking, and then closes her eyes and concentrates while taking each quarter inch, telling him that she won't choke and that he can take it out at any time. All she has to do is rise slowly. Every man's male identity is different, and each has sensitive spots and preferred ways of being handled. All a woman has to do is pay attention to her lover's needs. The sounds he makes and the feel of his body tensing are the best clues that she's doing it right. She should grasp with the hands the parts of the male identity that cannot fit into the mouth. Many men like as much stimulation as possible, and the feeling of a wet mouth and a moist hand is enough to send them to an orgasm very quickly.

She Should Know

She should find a position that works for both her and her partner. She should tell her partner what she likes and ask what they like—either before or during sex.

PERFECTING HER ORAL SKILLS

Here is the good news: it's easy to learn how to be a terrific penis handler. It does not matter the setting. It can be at home, in bed, or parked in the driveway. All that's needed is privacy.

Let's say the woman is on a couch. She has played, fondled, and warmed him up. She wants to give him a good blowjob; she slips down between his legs, opens his fly, and reaches in and touches his male identity. If he is hot for her, he will already be hard. If he is nervous or uninterested, it may still be bent up inside his shorts.

She takes hold of his male identity, leans toward his face, and kisses him. Is there a response down below? Any movement is a good sign. Now she pulls it out and sees how it stands. If it is stiff and sticking straight up or straight out, that's great. If it's wobbly or limp, she should do the following:

❦ Pull his testicles out. If his pants are too tight, pull them down. Now hold his testicles in the left hand and his male identity in the right. Squeeze it gently down toward the bottom of the shaft and get ready to suck it. Run the tongue over the lips to moisturize them and look into his face. He will want to watch her please him orally. Men love to watch.

❦ Open the mouth slightly to tease and excite him and come very close to his male identity. Breathe on him with her hot breath. Then, stick the tongue out again and reach for him, touch him, and tease him with it.

❦ Making sure the tongue is very wet, begin at the bottom of his shaft and slowly lick upward, turning her head sideways as if to take a bite of him. Slowly and gently, place the teeth onto his flesh. Wet him again using the tongue to help moisten him. A wet male identity looks and sounds a lot sexier than a dry one. Take the left hand and massage his family jewels, perhaps rubbing them ever so lightly with her fingernail bottom. The bottom will not hurt him, but the tips often do.

❦ Reach behind and underneath his family jewels to touch the sensitive area just before his anus, or run the fingers over his anus very lightly. Because the muscles that cause erection originate here, it will produce a reaction in his male identity.

❦ After she has licked his male identity a few times, getting it wet and hard, he will start squirming with frustration if the serious pleasure doesn't get started. A quick look up at his face will let her know if the teasing is too much. Having experience in giving blowjobs is a great education. She will know when that point has been reached.

❦ Do an upward swing with the tongue, from the base of his shaft to the rim of his knob. Continue long, moist licks over the top of his male identity. Linger at the hole in the center;

stick the tongue into it, if possible, but do not suck the head yet. Save for that later.

- Run the tongue around the rim of his knob, making frequent passes on the tender skin directly facing her. This is where most men are the most sensitive. One good thing to learn is that each man is unique and so is his male identity.

- Squeeze the shaft and see if some clear liquid drips out. If it does, dip the tongue into it and pull away. It will stretch with her and look fantastically erotic to her lover. Closing her eyes helps if she does not like the look of slimy things, because that's what it will look like.

- Act as if she loves it. Close in on his male identity head like it was chocolate ice cream and take the whole knob into her mouth. Hold it there. Listen to him moan. It will drive him crazy, and that is good.

- Now go down quickly and take his male identity into her mouth. Do not worry—it will not cause choking. If she bends the neck in just the right way, she can take it clear into the throat.

- Stay there, with the male identity down the mouth, for just a moment. Feel it inside the mouth. It can be as luscious as having one in the vagina. It grows on a woman.

- At this point, slide back up to the tip of the male identity and flick the tongue against it. Her man will be getting antsy now, wanting her to deep-throat him some more. However, she should not let him be a bully. If he had his way, it would all be over in two minutes, and that is no fun for her.

- Slide up and down on his male identity as if having inter-course. If he gets too close to coming, stop or at least slow down. If it is difficult to get all the way down to the bottom of his male identity, cheat a little by using the right hand to complete the sensation of deep throating him. It will look and feel as if she has the whole thing in the mouth. Slide the fingers, make an *O*-shape around the shaft, and then go up and down with the rhythm of sucking.

🦋 While mouthing the male identity, suck it, which feels quite different. There are deep sucks and little ones, and both feel great. He might have an idea of what he likes, so she should pay attention to his reactions. Taking just the knob in her mouth, suck it as if it were a nipple or a straw. This feels good to him, and he will get hot just thinking about it.

🦋 Now, take the whole male identity and suck it all the way up like a popsicle and then go back and do it again, sucking on the way down.

🦋 Any of these moves will feel great the first few times, but after a while, the male identity gets immune to feeling. When she senses this, she should move on to the next play. She does not ever want the male identity to go to sleep while she is in charge of it. She wants it to be constantly stimulated, but not quite to the point of orgasm, which is just about where she is now.

🦋 Okay, she has a raging hard-on in her right hand and some tight family jewels in her left. Lean back and look at them. Move the right hand all the way to the base of the male identity and squeeze it there. This will cause the shaft to fill and thicken, and by now his knob will be shining and smooth. Take the male identity into her mouth and suck it. Try various moves until he cannot stand anymore and he's ready to have an orgasm.

🦋 Allow his warm, wonderful juices to gush upward and slide the hands around his wet male identity. It will feel slippery and delightful to touch! Run the hands on it, feeling his hard male identity all the way to the top, smoothing the glistening fluids over his knob. This makes a great image for the woman and the man. He loves watching her play.

HER REFINEMENT

❦ There is one further refinement to this basic technique, which will heighten his orgasm. If she places the thumb at the base of his male identity in such a way as to block the tube, his semen cannot escape even though he is spasming and going through the reflex action of ejaculating semen.

❦ At the same time she sucks vigorously on the head of his male identity, delaying his cum for several moments. When she finally allows his semen to spurt, it will last longer and will be more intense for him. Even though the semen is delayed for a few short moments, he will be happy with the intensity of his semen spouting.

❦ She should not be so caught up in pleasing him that she misses out on her self-discovery. She should find out what works for both and make the sucking as individual as her signature. After all, she wants him to be able to clearly pick her out in the dark among hundreds of slobbering penis suckers.

Give him head that he will never forget and she will not be able to get rid of him. One woman in every fifty knows how to give a good blowjob. The rest act as if they are doing him a big

> **She Should Know**
>
> To get around a penis-induced gag reflex, try fake yawning.

favor. If the woman does not like to give a blowjob or she has hasn't learned to like it, she shouldn't give up. Maybe she will like it more as she grows older and becomes more sexually experienced.

Men feel that older women are much better at giving a blowjob. As the author of this book, I should warn women there are many women who like to give their men blowjobs. I have met many women who can have full-blown orgasms by simply sucking the male identity. Men know if one woman will not do it, there is always another woman out there who is willing. Some women just love to do it.

APPLYING PROPER SUCKING TECHNIQUES

The sad fact is that most women do not have the slightest idea of how to suck a male identity properly. Many women seem to think that simply making a circle with their mouth, closing it around a man's male identity, and bobbing their heads up and down until he climaxes. They think this will automatically makes her an expert sucker. Not true, my friends!

She should take the opportunity to look at and examine his male identity. Exploring each area of the male identity will help her find the most sensitive parts. Parts are parts, but some parts are more sensitive than others.

Let us discuss some great sucking techniques that are probably the most common male identity–sucking techniques in the world. In order for a woman to observe the man's reactions and get the most from his responses, she should:

- ❦ Take his male identity in the mouth, but not deeply. She should slide her moistened tongue lovingly over the head until the lips are closed around the shaft at the point just behind the corona. Do not just open the mouth and close it around his male identity; slide him in. He will enjoy it much more. Encase the shaft of his male identity with the hands. Remember the shaft is relatively insensitive to any kind of stimulation. Enclosing his male identity with the hands gives him the pleasurable sensation of having his male identity encased.

- ❦ Try twisting her head from side to side, making sure the moist lips stay in contact with his coronal ridge. While doing this, gently move the hands up and down his shaft. Gently suck around the corona as he climaxes to intensify his pleasure and increase the force of his orgasm. As she gains more experience, she will be able to tell exactly when his climax is approaching, and she will be ready for that initial spurt of satisfaction.

❦ While his erect male identity points toward the ceiling, cup his family jewels in one hand and carefully lick along the entire underside of his erect organ. While doing this, notice the areas that give him the most pleasure when the tongue is touching them. He will usually provide very vivid clues as to which areas are most pleasurable to him.

❦ Once she discovers the areas he likes to have caressed, concentrate more on those areas. For most men, the most sensitive area will be the point where the ring (or corona) of the head and the foreskin are attached, or where it was attached prior to circumcision. By licking and tapping along this area with the tongue, she will ensure that he arrives at ecstasy. To please him in a hurry, try to excite him in this way until he climaxes.

❦ When he is ready for climax, note the changes in his male identity. The head of the male identity may swell somewhat larger than it does during the normal course of his erection. He may thrust his hips forward as he wants to send his male identity inside her. For most men, immediately prior to orgasm there will be a clear drop or two of fluid at the tip of the male identity. When this happens, he is ready to have an orgasm.

Because of the structure of his male identity—as well as the structure of her mouth, lips, tongue, and teeth—a woman can provide a high degree of sensation to her lover and herself. She kneels between his legs and approaches his male identity from the bottom rather than from the side or the top. They should try various positions just to see what works best for her and him. It is usually a matter of personal preference.

A woman should place his stiff male identity inside her mouth but should not tighten her lips around the shaft. She should begin a circular motion with the head. The circle should be executed in both clockwise and counterclockwise motions in a slow, purposeful manner. The male identity will slide to different places in the mouth as the circular motion is continued. She should be careful—teeth are not allowed.

A kneeling position will suffice, but it is also effective when he is on his back and her head is directly over his male identity. When the technique is performed correctly, both can expect many hours of unadulterated pleasure.

GETTING RID OF THE GAG REFLEX

One of the first things a woman encounters when she starts to suck the male identity is the gag reflex. Some men want to force their male identity down her throat as far as they can get it, particularly at the moment they start to come.

The laws of nature seem to dictate that getting the entire male identity into a woman's mouth is impossible. A woman should not fret! It can be done. The biggest obstacle to taking his entire male identity down her throat is the fact that there is a bend of almost ninety degrees behind the tongue leading down into the throat. Therefore, the first thing to do is get the male identity past that angle.

GETTING PAST THE ANGLE OF HIS DANGLE

A woman must not allow her partner to get carried away at the moment he starts to climax. He will try his best to thrust his penis down her throat if he is inexperienced. She continues to relax the throat completely while he is thrusting deeply. It may require practice for her to take him completely. If she cannot, he will understand that this is not a rejection of him.

But she should not give up on mastering the deep-throating technique. She just keeps practicing and perfecting. If she desires to do it, she will ultimately succeed in deep-throating. In order to do this, she gets in a position where her head is turned in such a way that her mouth and throat lie almost in a straight line. The best way to accomplish this is for her to lie in bed so that her head is near the edge, with his body sprawled across the bed and her head tipped sharply back. This position will put her mouth and throat in a line and will allow her lover to approach her in such a way that insertion of his male identity is so deep that his pubic hair presses against the lips.

To get past the angle of his dangle, she should do the following:

🐏 Deep-throating. The natural tendency is to gag when a foreign object such as a deeply thrusting male identity is being forced down her throat. She can overcome this by completely relaxing the throat at the moment of insertion. It's equally important to maintain this relaxation during the entire deep-throating.

🐏 Practice with him. The man can now place his male identity down her throat and hold it still until he finds the most comfortable way to proceed. He's in full control and must initiate and maintain all the motion. He will relish this moment because it's the first time he can insert his male identity as deeply down her throat as he wants. Because of the position, she will not be able to move or offer him any greater stimulation than simply keeping her mouth tightly closed around his throbbing male identity. Try to stimulate the underbelly of his male identity with the tongue. All it takes is continuous practice.

꙳ Trust him. When a woman completely trusts a man, she's able to relax. This is the only exercise in which she relinquishes control of the situation to her lover. Trust him enough to enjoy the pleasure.

She Should Know

Edible, flavored lubrication gels are great for increasing the enjoyment of oral sex.

TESTICLES AND LOVEMAKING

Testicles are another portion of the male anatomy that should not be ignored in oral sex. The terms *family jewels, balls, testicles,* and *sacs* all describe the same part of the male identity. These are two male-owned objects that can enhance sensual feelings for men. Many people do not think of the jewels as primary sexual objects. They are extremely sensitive, and there must be a certain amount of trust before a man allows a woman to have undisputed use of his family jewels!

A woman should begin to play with the man's jewels, gradually increasing or decreasing the intensity as she gauges how he is responding. She should gently caress his male identity with her hand while she is bathing his family jewels with her tongue.

Because his family jewels are extremely sensitive to pain, a man will lose trust in a woman who does not respect the limits he places on them. She has the same right to place limits on the back of her throat until she is completely ready to receive him in her mouth, and he should be able to do the same with his family jewels.

Giving and Receiving

She should do it slowly and steadily. Anticipation is a great climax builder. She should make out with her partner for longer periods of time before going for the oral sex.

Once a man trusts a woman to take his jewels in her mouth, he will be more receptive to letting her wet them with her tongue prior to taking them into her mouth. Wetting the hairs down along the surface of the sac will keep her from causing pain to him. Women will discover an entirely new world of pleasurable sensations for her man when she takes the time to get to know his jewels

BECOME BETTER AT WHAT SHE DOES

Because there will be times she will want to satisfy him in a hurry, she should practice other oral lovemaking skills. He will enjoy spending time with her if she has sensuous tricks for him.

One trick is to place her lips around the head of his male identity and twirl them wetly and gently around the coronal ridge at the back of the penile head of his male identity. This skill will help him climax at a quicker rate. This does not require any great male identity–sucking skills, and it works because this is the area that is most sensitive on the man's body.

It is not necessary to be a perfect male identity sucker. All she has to do is to find the most sensitive area around the coronal area and focus on it continuously. It can produce a quick, powerful climax. She does not have to bob her head up and down on his male identity to get him off. Another use of this technique is to get him hard again after he climaxes so that he'll be rip-roaring to go again.

She Should Know

The frenulum is the spot where the glans meets the shaft on the underside of the penis just below the head, and the concentration of nerve endings here are compared to clitoris on a female.

DOING IT WELL REPEATEDLY

A woman should not be surprised if she finds herself wanting to go back for more. After she has satisfied her man, she should concentrate on a variety of techniques to get him excited again—not just to get him hard, but also to keep him hard enough to climax again! Sucking alone is not enough to satisfy him. She will need to combine the techniques she has learned with her own basic sucking techniques to stimulate him for a second and third time.

To help her accomplish this, she should explore his body: earlobes, neck, nipples, family jewels, anus, armpits, fingers, toes all those erotic areas that she missed while concentrating on his male identity. She should remember to include the navel, back of his neck, eyes, and any other parts of his body that might tickle him. It is important for her to explore his body and really get to know what makes him tick. She should not simply focus on his delightful male identity the entire time! When she explores, she is becoming a true male connoisseur.

SHE IS WHAT SHE EATS

Macrobiotic nutritionists have actually done research on this subject, and the answer is in: she is what she eats. Common sense dictates that if she tastes good, her lover will want to indulge in oral sex more often, so improving her body's taste and smell should be important to her.

In general, nutritionists say that alkaline-based foods, such as meats and fish, produce a buttery fish taste. Dairy products contain high bacterial putrefaction, creating the foulest-tasting fluids by far. But there is one food worse than dairy when it comes to how body fluids taste—asparagus. No one can miss the taste of asparagus-laced vaginal juices. Acidic fruits, sweets, and alcohol give bodily fluids a pleasant, sugary flavor, so she should eat lots of them so that she will more delicious than she already is.

Chemically processed liquors will cause an extremely acidic taste. So, if she wants to drink alcohol, she should choose high-quality, naturally fermented beers.

Giving and Receiving

The crease where the top of his thigh meets his butt is a surefire passion point. It's a sensitive area and could be the reason some people like being spanked.

SWALLOWING SEMEN

While he fantasizes about her swallowing his semen, mainly because pornographic movies display it as some kind of hero's badge of honor, some women find its taste or consistency difficult to swallow. It is a tricky situation, and men feel that if she swallows his semen, she accepts him completely. And, of course, if she loves her partner, she won't hurt his feelings by denying him this luxury. If the idea of swallowing turns her off, then doing it will not make the experience any more pleasurable. Fortunately, there is a way to swallow without really swallowing so that she and her partner are happy with the results.

> **She Should Know**
>
> Semen is so full of nutrients, it's a wonder people don't eat more of it.

A woman shows enthusiasm and lets her partner know that she is enjoying it. When she notices signs that he's about to come (he begins to pump faster, his breathing gets faster, and she begins to feel the initial contractions at the base of his penis), she pushes the back of her tongue up against the roof of her mouth, protecting the back of her throat and the sensitive taste buds. That way when he ejaculates, the fluids will pool in the front of her mouth. While the penis is still in her mouth, she slowly allows the semen to flow out of the side of her mouth and onto the back of her hand. Later she can discreetly wipe her hand on the sheets or a waiting towel. He will never know the difference. It will be her little secret.

EJACULATORY CALORIES

The question of semen content arises among persons who regularly swallow semen and who are concerned about calorie intake and nutritional substances.

Ejaculate is made up of many substances: fructose, lactic acid, ascorbic acid, blood-group antigens, sorbitol, calcium, chlorine, urea, cholesterol, choline, citric acid, creatine, deoxyribonucleic acid (DNA), glutathione, vitamin B12, hyaluronidase, inositol, magnesium, nitrogen, phosphorus, potassium, purine, pyrimidine, pyruvic acid, sodium, spermidine, spermine, uric acid, and zinc. The caloric content of ejaculate is approximately fifteen calories. Wow, who would have known this?

WHY MEN CRAVE ORAL PLEASURE

The more a man is feeling disconnected, the more he will crave sexual stimulation and release. The intensity of release at every stage of the sexual experience allows him to connect quickly with his feelings and his heart.

For him, sex is the experience of sexual pleasure and love. Although he may not be aware of it, his persistent sexual need is really his soul seeking completeness. As his need to be touched is satisfied, his ability to feel is also satisfied. When his feelings are awakened, his energy is freed. Through pleasure, he feels joy, love, and peace.

HER ORAL SEX GAMES

Some women get disappointed with their own lack of oral sex knowledge. With some patience and practice, anyone can be a fantastic licker, or oral lover. To become a great oral lover, a woman can.

1. Use cough drops. The next time she decides to give head to him, suck on a cough drop for a few seconds to get the mentholated twist working in her mouth. The heat from her tongue, the warmth of her breath, and the coolness from the cough drop give him a hot and cold sensation all at once. It will drive him erotically crazy. During oral sex, lightly blow on the male identity as it is sucked. This will help him keep a very nice and stiff erection. She does not have to suck the entire cough drop. About ten to twelve sucks are efficient. Save the

best sucking for his male identity. Continue this thrill until he begs for mercy. Remember to vary the moves.

2. Treat his male identity like a lollipop. Make circles around his male identity as she goes up and down on it. He will beg for mercy. Caress his inner thighs, buttocks, anus, tummy, and other parts of his body.

3. Lick his testicles gently. Take them into the mouth. This creates sensational pleasures for him. Move the tongue up and down, side to side in slow, lavishing licks. This is one of the most erotic pleasures to men, and not many women know it.

4. Play the sprinkle game. It is sucking at its very best and can get heated. Sprinkle tiny suction kisses all over his body. Begin from his head and work all the way down his entire body, stopping at his toes, then finally coming back up to his male identity. Now slip the tongue over all the areas that were just kissed, circling his eyes, ears, and lips. When she gets to his nipples, she can circle faster than before like a whirlpool. Pull his nipple into the mouth with suction kisses, pulling as much of his entire breast into the mouth as possible. Knead his nipples and gently pull them again. Suck him with pleasure and enjoyment as if trying to suck for taste.

5. Master the popsicle lick. A woman can use the tongue to circle the male identity clockwise. Slide the tongue in and out of the mouth and go counterclockwise. Add more thrills and sensations as she slides his male identity in and out, up and down. Go slow and speed up, then go slowly again. This sensuous lick has dramatic effects on a man and is worth every minute to see the effects. An added joy is working him over as if licking a favorite dessert.

6. Use the teeth as props. Hold his male identity sideways, like a buttered ear of corn. Slide the teeth gently up and down

his shaft. Giving it a gentle little nip every now and then is a fantastic blowjob.

7. Incorporate fruit. It's an added treat when accompanied with good oral sex. Bananas, oranges, berries, cherries, and any other luscious fruits are eaten as an appetizer to oral sex. Rubbing the juices all over his male identity and licking it off will send many sensations all over his body.

8. Try mint-flavored candies. Mouthwashes or breath mints create cool sensations.

9. Shake her head. Holding his male identity into the mouth, she gently shakes her head from side to side. This will send little tingles up and down his spine and throughout his male identity.

10. Alternate the mouth and vagina. This is stroke dipping. Men love this and tend to desire this one if the woman is open to it.

11. Make him more comfortable. Kneel down beside him and take his male identity in the palm of the hand while running the lips slowly over his male identity. She uses her tongue to circle his male identity head so that it simultaneously wets it and her own lips. She then opens her mouth and stretches her lips so that they cover the top and bottom rows of her teeth. Covering her teeth will help avoid nicks, bites, or cutting of his foreskin. Covering her teeth forms a smooth, firm ridge that creates highly sensitive sensations to the male identity. Place the male identity into her mouth down to the base and then come slowly back up.

12. Wet it. To keep sufficient lubrication for the male identity and to easily slide it in and out of her mouth, wet it a few times with her tongue.

13. Vary the speed. Be aware of the speed and remember to get in tune with his body movements. Study what sensations make him squirm, wiggle, or yell out, and then concentrate on these sensations. He might like slow, steady, continuous in-and-out motions, or he might prefer strong, quick strokes, or both. She should know what her man likes. Practice oral sex manipulations on a regular basis and before she knows it, he'll also know.

14. Give him a thrill. Take his male identity and move it gently between the lips. Hold it with the fingers while pressing its sides with the lips. Gently push it a little farther into the mouth and forcefully suck it in and out as far as it will go. Now press the end of his male identity against the roof of the mouth. Suck it deeply as if trying to swallow him. He will experience ecstasy.

15. Surprise him. As he watches TV or listens to music, she can innocently unzip him and suck away to her heart's content.

16. Complete the eat. A loving and sexy thing to do is to lavishly ingest his penile juices after he's had his orgasm. It is a fantastic topper to sexual encounters.

17. Exercise the tongue. Want to give the most amazing oral sex ever? Exercise the tongue in front of a mirror twice a day. Point the tongue and push it forward, then flicker it from side to side, keeping a smooth and steady rhythm. Try to touch the nose and chin with smooth and steady motions.

> **She Should Know**
>
> If a man has an inactive sex life, sperm that stores up inside his body without begin released will eventually die and be reabsorbed into his body like horse manure spread judiciously throughout a cornfield.

18. Give gentle kisses on his male identity. Try it in a dark restaurant. Sneaking is fun. Do it under a table. Make sure the table is dressed in a floor-length cloth to provide secrecy.

A NOTE FOR HER

Fellatio is performed with enthusiasm. She loves what she is doing to him, either because she loves him or she loves sucking his male identity. Loving both is best! Faked orgasms have nothing on lackluster fellatio, which is one of the worst things a woman can do to a man.

A NOTE FOR HIM

A man should never push it. There is nothing more deadly than having a man push a woman's head down toward his male identity. If she is into it, she will come around to it, but sometimes not until the second time she makes love with him. Whatever the case may be, do not force it. If she takes her time, she will learn to like it. If she does not enjoy it, perhaps his next lover will.

At a certain time in every girl's life,
she understands that men are visual creatures.

Chapter 18

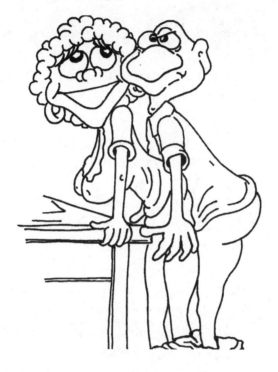

Her Gratifying Tune-Ups
(aka Quickies)

There is nothing more exciting than a session of slow leisurely sex,
but on occasion, a quickie is what the doctor ordered.

Sexual tune-ups make the man feel good because there are no restrictions or feelings of rejection. Not being rejected makes him feel passionately attracted to his partner. Not feeling pressure makes the woman feel more loved, which encourages her to want to have more sex freely and willingly. Because of quickies, a woman stops feeling pressured to have sex. She now feels that she is getting the kind of sex she wants and is in return giving him the kind he wants.

Women and men can work as a team to reduce the time it takes to have good sex. When time is short, they choose to skip foreplay and move right into sexual intercourse. Just about every man experiences those times when he just wants to take his woman, have his sexual way with her, and then get on with the day without having to go through the entire foreplay and after-play process.

Of course, there is nothing wrong with wanting a little quickie sex on occasion; believe it or not, there are plenty of women who enjoy it hard and fast and without all that fluffy stuff. The reality is that a woman has to know how to go about enjoying quickie sex without a man making her feel like he is about to leave a crisp twenty on the nightstand. When a woman really trusts the man, something deep down inside her wants to cut loose and completely let go without any restraint or worry of "nice girls don't do that" kind of thinking. She wants to be free and feel free while making love. She would like to make her partner happy, but she wants to experience happiness too. A sexual tune-up gets that done quickly. She wants the kind of sex most women refer to as a quickie. Women affectionately use the term *tune-up* as in sexual tune-up. It is a grown woman's term.

> **She Should Know**
>
> A quickie is one of the best ways to make sure she still gets between-the-sheets—even if only for a few minutes. The reality of having a great sex life filled with sensual lovemaking sessions can be difficult to pull off. Stealing away five or ten minutes is totally doable.

SHE WANTS AND NEEDS A TUNE-UP

Did I really say that? Women, for whatever reason, must have a sexual tune-up from time to time.

There is nothing more exciting than having a session of slow, leisurely sex, but on occasion, she just doesn't have time or energy for the marathon sex, and sometimes even prolonged sex is not what she wants. A quickie may be just what the doctor recommends.

It is not that she does not want to bump and grind with her man for long periods, but sometimes she just wants to be sexed. She wants it when she wants it, as soon as she feels the urge. She does not want to hold back because at that particular time, all she needs is to get her freak on, and she does not want to spend a lot of time doing it.

> **She Should Know**
>
> Quickies are not meant to remove sensuality and intimacy. Kissing is always a great way to start the intimacy and keep it going. She shouldn't negate the important aspects of physical connection. Quickies are about both partners.

Sometimes a woman wants good loving from a good man without all the pre-sex commotion. Quickies are great for every sexually active couple. The man can follow the woman's lead occasionally, without being told when and how to revel in the freakiness of it all.

When a man knows what to do, how to do it, and when to do it, he then knows what needs to be done to turn a woman on. He knows that she does not want to talk about it or direct his actions, she just wants a good screwing to let go of her inhibitions and express herself, and she wants it done right.

HER GUILT-FREE QUICKIES

Feeling the need to be sexed and acting on it is difficult for many women because they have been groomed since childhood to think differently. Let us look at the following scenario: Ricky always felt a little guilt after having sex with Rosilyn because it was evident that she was not satisfied. Ricky felt that foreplay was what she wanted, and if he did not give it to her, he felt that he had cheated her. To combat this, they would always wait until it was bedtime to have sex because it felt right not rushing it. Rosilyn wanted some quickies though. She would suggest sex right before it was time for the children to come home so she could have a tune-up, but it did not always work out. He wanted to give foreplay, and she only wanted a tune-up. Her quickies made her feel guilt free, but he felt like he was shorting her. They just could not get it together. After beating themselves up for a while about their timing problems, they decided to negotiate.

Rosilyn told Ricky that she wanted more sexual encounters that were spur of the moment. She did not need foreplay before sex each time. She asked him what she could do to make him feel better about having more guilt free tune-ups.

Ricky felt that if Rosilyn only wanted a tune-up, the passion in their relationship would die out. Rosilyn felt that if all Ricky wanted were long sexual escapades (gourmet sex), they would never have time for sex. They compromised about taking turns initiating their special kind of sex and decided to have a romantic getaway at least once a month where both of them could indulge in each other's sexual wishes.

Rosilyn loved tune-ups, and Ricky preferred gourmet sex, so they decided to have both. Rosilyn promised Ricky more pleasure, loving attention, and pampering, and he promised her more pleasurable quickies.

STAYING COMMITTED TO THE TUNE-UP

Let's start by answering a few questions. Are a woman's sexual tune-ups simply a temporary Band-Aid, or do her tune-ups make her feel better for longer periods? Is it like fast food that she enjoys when woofing it down, or is it the long-term fulfillment of her sexual needs? She should never do anything that makes her feel uncomfortable emotionally, physically, or sexually. Making time for sex begins with a woman's personal journey into her own sexuality and sexual attitude. There are several ways women can have regular sex.

- ❦ Fast food sex: sexual tune-ups (aka quickies)
- ❦ Gourmet sex: longer session with foreplay
- ❦ More affection: regular love attention with hugs and kisses
- ❦ Sexual getaway: at least once a month

With a tune-up, her anticipation is heightened because she knows she is going to have sex. When tune-ups are incorporated into the regular sexual routine, the man and the woman both feel free to have the kind of sex they desire. This newfound sexual freedom recharges a man's sex life and energizes a woman's. A woman really does want sex, but she needs to feel the man's emotional support. More than anything else, she needs to feel needed.

CHANGING HER ATTITUDE ABOUT SEX

Women will never reach a higher level of sexual awareness if they do not change their attitudes about sex. Women often think that sex is done in the dark or kept under wraps. For some it is alluring, and to others it is questionable rather than pleasurable. Some women use sex to cure their ills for the moment: loneliness, boredom, anger, and depression.

No act can be quite so intimate as the sexual embrace.

~Havelock Ellis

Chapter 19

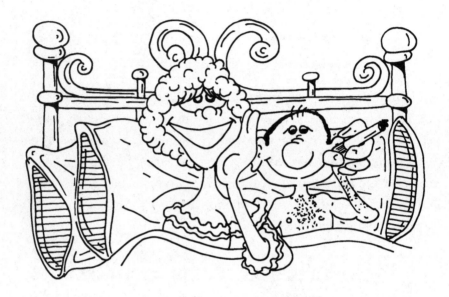

Her Good Sex

A good sex life is a major factor in creating pleasure.

The popular question is when does a woman's sensuality allow her sexuality to take over? It all begins with the woman, but it continues when she is with her man. Sexuality starts when she looks into his eyes. In order for a woman to capture a man's heart, she's got to first catch his eye. Every woman has this gift! It does not matter how young, old, tall, short, thin, wide, dumb, smart, rich, poor, good, or bad—everyone serves a divine purpose in this life, which includes taking care of the self, attracting love and living a good life.

Even if a woman dates on the internet, the relationship begins with her eyes. Observe what catches a woman's eyes when she first meets a man in whom she is interested. Is it his physical aspects? Is it his conversation? Is it plain ol' female curiosity? She might think to herself, *Hmmmmm, he is not a bad-looking person, but will he want to meet me?* While a woman continues to evaluate herself under the scrutiny of her own microscope, men see her quite differently than she sees herself. She sees that he has that "something," and he sees that she has that "thing!" Because beauty is in the eye of the beholder…to each of them, it's all good.

SHE'S GOT THAT THING

Every man has a favorite thing about a woman that he cannot resist. It may be her physical aspects, her personality, or her character. It might be several factors, but a woman wants all her features to be just right. That's why a woman is so hard on herself. She is trying to make sure she has what he wants. She puts in lots of time and effort in becoming this so-called perfect woman for him, but what she does not realize is… she already has what he wants and likes. It is *that thing* she has, some might say. She catches his eye because there is something about her he likes, even though neither of them knows what it is. They cannot quite explain it, but they know it's there. It is inside his head, but he does not know how to put it into words yet. It might be that thing she does, or that thing she says while walking, talking, standing, sitting, or simply being who she is. It is just that thing! Whatever that thing is, it will hold his gaze until she snaps her finger.

HER HEATED PLEASURES

A heated sex life is not just the symptom of a passionate relationship; it is also a major factor in creating pleasure. Pleasure fills most couples' hearts with love. It can fulfill almost all our emotional needs. But heated sex, loving sex, passionate sex, sensual sex, long sex, short sex, quickie sex, gourmet sex, playful sex, tender sex, rough sex, soft sex, hard sex, romantic sex, goal-oriented sex, erotic sex, simple sex, compli-cated sex, cool sex, and hot sex are each an important part of keeping passion alive.

> **She Should Know**
>
> She should focus on inti-macy. True intimacy involves listening to the other person and opening up about what she's thinking and feeling.

Without passion, sex is routine and boring. By combining heated sex skills with love, a couple can continue to experience great passion and fulfillment. Instead of becoming less passionate over the years, a woman who sees and touches her lover's naked body can become turned on more than ever. Not only does she become excited by the pleasure of arousal and increasing sexual intensity, she becomes aware of how much more love, warmth, passion, and sensual affection she can experience and provide for him. This awareness elevates sex to a higher level of passion, excitement, and commitment.

When a woman feels passion for a man, he can rejoice in her continued desire to connect with him and provide her lasting plea-sure. She is the one who recognizes sex as an opportunity to share her gentleness and love in a way that nurtures him the most. Sex becomes a beautiful expression of her love for him and an opportunity to receive his love.

Sex is fabulous when shared in love. Sex gives love a chance to grow. For a woman to grow in sexual fulfillment, she needs to feel successful in fulfilling her sexual needs. She should not be afraid to try new skills in her relationship or bed.

PLEASURE OPENS HER HEART

A woman's heated pleasure allows her to become softer and gentler in spirit. The love in her heart is open, and she is more willing to accept love from her partner. Her partner's skillful and knowing touch leaves no doubt in her mind that she is important to him. The hunger for love is fulfilled with her partner's passionate and present attention. Tension is released as she surrenders to the deepest longings of her feminine being; her passion to love and be loved is fulfilled.

HER PLEASURE OPENS HIS SOUL

A man's heated pleasure helps him release his frustrations and allows him to rekindle his passion and commitment to the relationship. It quickly helps him experience positive results for his efforts.

In an intimate relationship, a woman's fulfillment is the ultimate quest of a man. Her warm and moist responses excite and awaken his male being. He feels as though the world is opening up to him. He feels appreciated through her fulfillment. He feels his desire as she returns in his world while remaining inside of her moistness. He loves the way it feels and smells, and how it thrills him. He wants to do it repeatedly.

When a man touches a woman and feels her softness, she begins to feel pleasures that he has longed for. Through touching, she can connect with his own kindness while he remains masculine and focused on taking care of her.

When connecting through sex, a man's soul is reawakened, allowing him a chance to understand why it is so important to feel pleasure again. Sex allows a man to connect with his feelings and his sensitivities. Many times, after having great sex, a man can regroup and regain insight on the beautiful things in life. He is more understanding and kinder in a hard world. He can breathe again and feel inner peace and joy. Sex is good for a man's soul.

She Should Know

She should own her sex life and try to get to know her own body better by exploring it with her hands or a handy vibrator.

KEEPING THE FIRES BURNING

When the home fires are burning, it reminds both the man and the woman of the highest love and heat that first brought them to one another. Heated sex generates the wonderful chemicals in the brain and body that allow the fullest enjoyment of one's partner. It increases the attraction for both partners as it stimulates energy and enthusiasm. It promotes better health practices and makes us appreciate each other for the big and small things. Heated sex helps people make sex and love a priority in their lives. How women mate, relate, and communicate has changed a great deal over the years, and so have sex skills. To fulfill her partner in bed, fresh skills are required. After a short while in any relationship, sex can sometimes become boring and routine. By making a few minor adjustments, women and men can completely overcome this problem.

She Should Know

She should schedule sex. By simply making sex a priority, she's not putting it on the back burner and hanging it out to dry.

IMPROVING HER SEX

Sex can always use improvement, but like anything else, it requires new information and the opportunity to practice. Most women are never taught how to have sex, but once they learn how to get turned on or masturbate, they are expected to be sexual experts. A woman knows how to help a man have an orgasm, but the art of great sexual fulfillment is a different story altogether.

For great sex, a woman needs to understand a man's body and what she can do to remain turned on as she pleases him. It is difficult for a woman to know what she needs to get turned on all the time. It is hard for men to know what turns a woman on and how to keep her happy in bed because each is expected to already know what the other one wants. She assumes that he knows how to make her happy, and he assumes that what makes him happy also makes her happy. When a woman isn't satisfied, a man thinks it's something wrong with her instead of his techniques. He does not accept or understand that her needs are tremendously different from his.

SHE LIKES IT SLOW, HE WANTS IT FAST

When a woman moves slowly during sex, she is trying to tell him that she wants nurturing. She wants her body to be massaged, not beat up. A man will not know what a woman likes unless she shows him. Even when she tells him, he forgets the next time they have sex. He is thinking more of what he wants than what she needs. Even though he knows she likes a slow grind, when he gets excited he speeds up. He thinks she wants it faster because that is what he wants. Women like slow penetration most times. If he is smart, he will know he should slow down to make her climb the walls to ecstasy every time they make love. Over time, both lovers discover how to fulfill each other's sexual needs.

LOSS OF HER SEXUAL DRIVE

Being sensuous, alive, and vibrant is vital to the success of a woman's inner spirit and her relationship. Women who have lost their sexual desire or sensuous drive grow old before their time. Loss of sexual appetite leads to frustration and the possible loss of a loving man.

When a woman loses the desire to make love or her interest in sex dies, she should start making plans to get in touch with her sensuous side. If she puts out undesirable messages to the man in her life, he soon begins to think that he is undesirable, unloved, and unwanted.

Many times, women who are no longer in a loving and romantic relationship send messages of being

> **She Should Know**
>
> She should play a sex game. If she has a hard time thinking of exactly how to make up crazy positions or how to change up foreplay, the retail world has her back. She can create fun, sensuous games both partners will love to indulge in.

a bitch. This is because these women are usually angry and uptight. They need some good loving. When she gets sex, she becomes a softer, kinder, and gentler person. When she does not, she appears angry at the world, and everyone around her tends to suffer.

WAYS TO ENJOY SEX

Many women enjoy sex. Some enjoy it some of the time, some enjoy it most of the time, and, unbelievably, there are women who enjoy sex all the time. Maybe these women even love it all, from the very thought of it to the afterglow. They have more sex than the rest of us, and they thrill their men to the core. Whether they are feeling hot for their lovers or just lukewarm, they would rather do it than not do it—they make love, not excuses.

What makes sex great is love. Getting to know someone better helps pleasure and love grow. The more sensual the experience, the more chance it has to thrive and become something positive. If she is tired, sex can revive her. If she is stressed, it relaxes her. And if she has a headache, instead of falling asleep, she opts for the orgasm cure. To help her achieve this, she should:

1. Plan and follow through on sex quotas. When both are juggling a hundred different things, finding time for a little loving might be the last thing on her mind. Make sure it is on the schedule and takes top billing. Assign a weekly sex goal. Every Monday, pick a random number and schedule time for sex that number of times before the weekend. If three days go by with zero action, make up the time fast. Get busy reaching the quota.

2. Crank up her sex drive. Sexual connoisseurs never sit around waiting for the mood to strike—they make the mood happen. Waiting for sex to happen in the midst of daily obligations means sex will become a very rare event. She will often

reminisce about the last time she had great sex—such as thinking about his touch, his warm breath on her skin, and his sweet murmurings in her ear. Focus on sexy moments that will bring about a fired-up state of mind. Think of those things that will lead her to the bedroom for some great sex.

3. Take turns giving and receiving. Many times, one of the lover's energy will not be tuned in to the same sex channel. This is the time one will have to decide who is going to be the giver and who will be the receiver. The energetic person should be the giver, and the one without a lot of energy should be the receiver. The giver ignites the fires, and the receiver allows the giver to do the turning on.

    ❦ There are going to be times when she will not have to raise a finger and can relax and enjoy the ride. It's guilt free because the giver knows the favor will be returned another night. Think of all those times he was denied sexual happiness because she was too tired to oblige him. Now she will have much happier sexual adventures because both are making an effort to keep their home fires burning.

4. Alternate the times she has sex. Her sex life will definitely suffer if the only time she has sex is by a set schedule. Get rid of the ideas that sex should be a nighttime ritual, and soon discover that there are plenty of times to indulge. Try different times—for instance, immediately after work, soon after happy hour, or weekend afternoons or midmornings. Have sex before leaving for work for guaranteed satisfaction.

5. Have a titillating soundtrack. Music has a way of altering people's moods in an instant, so it comes as no surprise that the right CD could steer lovers straight to the bedroom. Play some romantic music to pump up the passion.

6. Consider pleasure as a cure-all. Excuses, excuses—it is so easy to find reasons to put off slipping into bed and making love. Exhaustion or stress, annoyance and bickering—stop right there and consider what is sexy. Divas know all too well that doing the deed can actually alleviate exhaustion, stress, and marital tension—the very things that are supposedly keeping her from having sex in the first place! Sex energizes rather than drains, so find plenty of opportunities to use a little loving for an energy boost. "Just do it"—she will be glad she did afterward. Think of sex as a way to connect and feel calmer rather than just another thing on a to-do list.

7. Be passionate all day. Do not reserve libidinous fervor just for the bedroom. Live out sexual happiness by adding spice to everyday activities. Wear silk undies. Buy an ice cream cone and eat it suggestively. Take the most luxurious shower before work with all sorts of wonderful scrubs and creams. These things keep erotic energy constant.

8. Keep the pleasure buzzing. Do things in the morning that will keep him lusting. Such gestures as stretching while naked; bending over while getting dressed; or raising the arms, arching the back, and sticking the chest out in front of him work wonders. Calling out to him in the morning from the shower to bring her a towel gives him sensuous ideas too. Give him hints to rerun in his mind. Sex is usually inevitable that evening.

9. Do not saddle sex with tons of work. Passionately prolific women have a philosophy: frequent sex, no matter what kind, is an absolute must for a good marriage. So if sex sometimes has to be a quickie—aka tune-up—so what? It's still good sex. If the kids are coming home from school in twenty minutes, do not try to light a bunch of candles and dig out the favorite

set of love songs. This is when the window of opportunity is short, so jump each other's bones in a hurry. It does wonders for the sex life and relationship.

10. Think about the pleasure of sex. Conventional wisdom and scientific research says that men think about sex more often than women do. Rather than censoring their erotic thoughts, some women encourage them. These women do not feel guilty about fantasizing, even if their fantasies are a bit kinky or feature some creative casting. And because sex is so often on their minds, it's a lot easier for their bodies to get to "yes."

11. Boost the libido. Indulge in sensuous thinking. One woman might be turned on by looking at a pile of luscious peaches and easily let her mind drift to imagine the fruit as her lover's balls. Another woman might think about her sexy lover and picture parts of him, like his forearm or chest, until she is highly aroused. However, even the most mundane things can have an erotic appeal. Something as simple as running her hand along a wooden stick shift in a car can become a sensuous experience. It's all in her mind.

12. Put sex at the top of the "things to do" list. Another positive way to get the sexual motor going is to make notes. Just like a grocery list, be sure to list sex as one of the favorite things to do. The note is there as a reminder. Make the notes interesting and fun. Here's an example of a simple but sexy note: "Make love on top of the pool table."

13. Take a mood and give it an erotic charge. Any emotion—even sadness—can be the catalyst for passion if there is an erotic connection. Learn to take the present mood and turn it into a sensual advantage. The positive result is better sex and a more passionate relationship.

14. Heal through pleasure and sex. For many women, the hardest part about being in a committed relationship is learning to share their emotions—all of them.

    ❦ It is easy to be happy with someone and more difficult to be sad. Many times when a man is feeling bad or shutting down the communication in a relationship, a woman can provide a little pampering and understanding, and help him heal through romance. Find erotic revelations in every emotion. Erotic interludes bring couples closer during times when intense emotion might drive a wedge between them.

15. Indulge in sensuality. Take pride in the thrill of the feel. Rub silk against his body. Women who love sex delight in all their senses. They breathe deeply of the flowers others merely sniff. They take pride in making love. Nothing makes a woman feel sexier than self-indulgence. Whether having her legs waxed or buying new makeup, lingerie, or a bag of very expensive chocolates to eat on the way home, an indulgence can make her feel pampered and sexy. No matter how busy she is, she should find time to schedule indulgence time. No husband, kids, friends, work—just pampering time. Send the kids to relatives for a couple of hours and relax in bed a little longer. Take private time to read a book, or hire a sitter and go to a midafternoon movie. Occasional time-outs can restore the body and rejuvenate the soul. It allows time to experience the interesting parts of her life. Self-indulgence becomes more intriguing.

16. Wear sexy, simple, elegant clothing and lingerie. Invest in camisoles. Wear them often beneath business suits. Wearing them feels sensuous and very sexy.

17. Never stop fantasizing. A woman often says, "I'm married, not dead," when she's trying to explain how she needs love and affection. Sex-loving women can relate to this statement

because they really adore men. They do not stop liking them once they take their marriage vows. They are married, not nuns. Women can respectively indulge in sexual fantasies, whether driving to work, riding an elevator, waiting in line, or pumping gas. A woman can weave little erotic stories around the men she encounters. She might imagine a construction worker with bulging biceps as her secret lover.

18. Flirt with her lover to keep the attraction alive. There is nothing wrong with flirting, but lighthearted flirting with a stranger, a coworker, or male friend can also get the juices going. An exchange of smiles, compliments, and flirty gestures with him will also make her feel more desirable.

19. Make the most of her body. Sex-loving women are not always the most beautiful women. They do not always have perfect measurements, either, but they like their bodies. Exercise in some form is generally a priority, not because they want to be thinner, but because they crave the physicality. They know how to use their bodies to excite their lovers. Working out gives a woman's body a sexy afterglow and helps prepare it for making love.

20. Never be afraid to touch herself. Women who love sex are comfortable with touching themselves. They are not afraid to masturbate. It's how they learn about their own bodies, about what they like and how they can reach orgasm quickly or slowly (depending on their mood). Since most women do not reach orgasm via intercourse alone, those who feel free to touch themselves during lovemaking control their erotic destiny. They know what they want, and that makes them more confident and relaxed lovers. When a woman knows that she can get up to speed quickly, it makes her more willing to

follow the man's lead. Even if she thinks she is not in the mood she can help get herself there with a little masturbation.

21. Expect her partner to be a good lover. Sex-loving women have high standards—for themselves and their lovers. They want to be good lovers, but they also want to get love as good as they give it. They know their men want to give them real orgasms. In addition, if a woman's lover needs gentle instruction in that regard, she is happy to provide it.

Many women lose interest in sex because their lovers become lousy lovers. Women read sex advice often; men rarely do. A woman should share new ideas with him and help him out.

Sex can get a man, but sex cannot keep a man.

Chapter 20

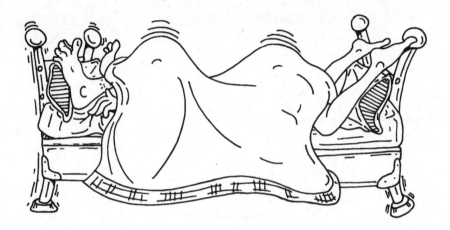

Her Gratifying Sex Treats

Being aware of what it takes to be a sensuous woman
is also being in tune with her wants and needs.

It can sometimes become difficult when a woman wants to release inhibitions and enjoy being a sexually sensuous woman. To achieve intense sensuous pleasures before, during, and after sex, she has to make contact that is more sensuous with her lover. She will feel comfortable in the relationship when she is able to loosen up, get rid of sexual hang-ups, and express her love. Mood and privacy are basic concerns, but she should also feel the environment is safe, romantic, and comfortable before it becomes completely erotic.

Giving and Receiving

She should create a sex bucket list. She should make a numbered list of things she and her partner want to try. Then, they should set a date for when they'd like to accomplish these goals by. What matters is the thrill of new places and moves to go with them.

Some women manage to keep their sensuality in full bloom long after their friends have thrown in the towel. A woman can get in tune with her sensuality and improve it if she is shown love and sincere appreciation. If she has lost interest in making love and cannot seem to get the hots for her lover, she is allowing her feminine sensuality to suffer. Maybe she is focused on the bills, family problems, or other nonsexual activities. Whatever it is, she should refocus and rediscover her sexual self so that she can get turned back on. Being aware of what it takes to be a sensuous woman is also being in tune with her wants and needs. To help her get the most from her heated moments, a woman can do the following:

1. Sit close and touch him sensuously as often as possible.

2. Stand next to him and stroke his back, moving the hands slowly and sensuously.

3. When at social gatherings, brush the nipples across his body each time he passes by.

4. Pull him closer when kissing. Do not allow him to be the aggressor every time.

5. Give long, lingering, and playful kisses. Feel the pleasure of the kiss by giving many tongue kisses.

6. Gliding the hips toward him while kissing, roll onto his male identity sensuously.

7. Play with his nipples each kiss.

8.   Do things that he likes.

9.   Blindfold him and make love to him. Become willing to share sensuous ideas with him.

10.   Look him directly in his eyes while he gets masturbated.

11.   Name a new dessert after his male identity.

12.   Place her forefinger into her vagina, and as she hugs him, give him a long sensuous kiss. Now slowly glide the vagina-scented finger under his nose.

13.   As she stares into his eyes, slowly and seductively suck on an ice cube. Move the ice cube in and out of the mouth with the tongue, and then release it from the lips, while licking the rim of the glass slowly and sensuously.

14.   Have him massage the love button with his penis.

15.   Wear something sexy to bed at least five times a week.

16.   Buy a garter belt and wear it with no panties. While he eats dinner, she can open and close her legs so that he can see her hungry vagina.

17.   Revamp by buying sexy matching bra and panty sets.

18.   Buy a vibrator and learn how to use it, and then teach him how to use it.

19.   Buy sheer stockings instead of support hose.

20.   Wear sexy laced bras regularly.

21.   Read sexual books to liven up sensuous thinking.

22.   Give good phone sex. Do not forget to coo and ahh a lot. Seduce him by making a sensuous call to him for a date.

23.   Hire him for an evening of passionate sex. Pretend to pay him a hundred dollars an hour. He will think about it all day.

24.   Tell him that he turns her on and mean it.

25.   Look good when he's at home from work. He probably sees beautiful women daily, some who probably flirt with him. Do not give him a reason to have an affair.

26.   Be a good listener when he talks. Look him in his eyes and listen to what he has to say.

27.   Think about sex with him on a regular basis—it makes her sexier.

28.   Work to be the best sexual lover he has ever had.

29.   Fulfill one of his fantasies.

30.   Schedule two fantasy dates per month. Both are responsible for one each. Keep all plans secret from each other.

31.   Plan an evening around a sexual fantasy. Make it as wild as possible. Make it a date to remember.

32.   While giving oral sex, take a piece of ice into the mouth. Slip his male identity into the mouth, rotate the ice cube all around it, making sure to lick and massage it with the tongue until he begs for mercy. This is very beneficial to a limp male identity.

33.   Tie him to the bed and tease him. Touch him with parts of her sensuous body only.

34.   After seductively stripping for him, kiss him all over his body, remembering not to miss a single spot. Alternate soft to firm touches on his body. As he squirms and twitches

about, leave him there and get a drink or find something else to do for about two minutes. These two minutes will feel like twenty to him. Come back to him and start the process over again beginning with light kisses on his body. It will drive him crazy.

35. Send items of sexy clothing to him. The schedule for sending these articles of clothing is up to her. For example, if she wants him to receive all items in one week, she sends everything at once. If she wants to prolong the anticipation over two weeks, she sends half this week and half the following week. This game is as sensuous and erotic or as subtle as the woman wants. Clothing should be sensuous and erotic. Once he receives the complete outfit, wear it for him.

36. Skinny-dip with him.

37. Give oral sex with a mouth full of ice-cold water.

38. Suck on a strong mint before performing oral sex.

39. Help him withdraw from intercourse just before the point of no return, going back to it soon after.

40. Slow down all movement just before he ejaculates. Move all body parts as if belly dancing very slowly.

41. Provoke a quickie. Strip naked for him while he keeps his clothes on.

42. Leave panties on during sex or have him tear the panties off to get to the sweet, awaiting vagina.

43. Make his male identity hard without touching it. Whisper softly that she wants to feel him inside of her and watch how it turns him on.

44. While placing his head over her heart and allowing him to listen to her heartbeat, tell him that he helps her live.

45. Ask him to pinch her nipple and watch it go from soft to hard. Tell him how hard she likes it to be done and make sure he reaches her hardness goal.

46. Place lipstick around the head of his male identity and suck it off slowly and gently, then give slower and harder suction actions.

47. Place a large rubber sheet on the floor. Coat his body with massage oil and then have a timed wrestling match. First to achieve two holds can ask the other for any sexual treat they desire. Coating the sheet with oil will add more escalated slippery fun.

48. Send him an e-card designed to tantalize and turn him on.

49. Hand-deliver any obscene messages. It's deemed illegal to send obscene letters through the mail.

50. Ask him to stay at the shallow end of the vagina during massaging thrusts as the outer third of the vagina is the most sensitive. Having him dip the tip of his male identity into her vagina feels great.

51. Do it in the cupboard under the stairs—seriously. Novelty is an intense aphrodisiac, and any unusual setting with strange sensations, smells, and muffled sounds will make sex feel new, upping the excitement.

52. Sit on top of the washing machine with the legs wrapped around his waist. Washing machine vibrations turns the male identity into a wonderful vibrator. Select the cotton cycle for best results. Pick a warm wash cycle so her butt

won't get cold, and make sure it has the longest, fastest spin. Feel the vibrations. She will want more once he does this.

53.   Place a pillow under her bottom to create an orgasm with optimum twenty-six-degree pelvic tilt, which means maximum contact between his body and her G-spot. This will help a woman reach orgasm every time.

54.   Have early-in-the-morning sex. Because hormones are at their peak during the morning, early morning sex is great. Try side-by-side sex or spoon away from each other. This way she doesn't have to worry about brushing her teeth or freshening her breath.

55.   Choose colors to create sexy moods. Red, dark blue, and violet are the three most erotic colors. And the least erotic is gray.

56.   Have sex in the bath. This is fun but also tricky. Try this: fill the bath halfway with water and then pour plenty of bath gel over each other's bodies. With her man lying down in the bath, lie on top of him and, instead of going for penetrative sex, stimulate each other to climax by rubbing bodies.

57.   Rotate the palms of the hands on areas near his male identity to build excitement.

58.   Pull a sexy piece of underwear from her drawer and ask that he wear it beneath his clothing.

59.   Plan a special dinner out. Choose sensuous appetizers and a main course. Plan a long meal, but remember to mention lots of suggestive, sensuous games and gestures. Make the suspense of what's going to happen later last as long as possible.

60. Take turns with the Tongue Joy Oral Vibrator. Strapped to the tongue, the vibrations stimulate nerve endings like never before.

61. Play Twister in the nude while wet. It removes inhibitions and gets her in positions she wouldn't usually attempt.

62. Don't go solo with the vibrator. Only 25 percent of women climax through penetrative sex alone, so get him to pleasure her with a sex toy while he is making love.

63. Ask him to talk or hum his favorite tune while he is indulging in oral sex. The vibrations from his voice and the unpredictability of it will make her come quicker.

64. Feed him cinnamon, cardamom, peppermint, or lemon if he is going to be treated to oral pleasure. It will make his semen taste nicer.

65. Convince him to buy you jewelry by masturbating him with a string of pearls. Use lots of lubrication and then wrap the pearls around the shaft of his male identity, gently sliding them up and down. They will add different levels of stimulation to the experience. He will love buying jewelry just to see what treats she has in store for him.

66. Remember the mind-blowing sex of yesterday. Today is a new day, so each lovemaking session should be new and eventful.

67. Do not be apologetic for her shape, size, or physical appearance. She should improve it if feels she has to apologize for any part of her body.

68. Be human. The human part of her means more than anything else.

69.   Leave a sexually suggestive message on his private voicemail.

70.   Refuse to be judged by other's standards. Share pleasure with him that might not be normal to others. It is her love life, hopefully no one else's.

71.   Wake up before he does and makes love until he climaxes.

72.   Play with him using honey until he climaxes.

73.   Ask him about his favorite sex techniques. Let him show her how he likes to do it.

74.   Take nude photographs of him playing with his private parts.

75.   Let him take pictures of her while she plays with her vagina.

76.   Make up a game called "find the balls," with his rules, and then play with them.

77.   Bite his butt cheeks gently from time to time during sex.

78.   Let him lick her all over until she climaxes.

79.   Greet him at the door wearing heels only.

80.   Serve him dinner stark naked, with her as the dessert.

81.   Let him trim her pubic hair.

82.   Watch him shave his pubic hair.

83.   Play with his male identity before he goes to work.

84.   Make passionate love to him before he goes to work.

85.   Catch him in the shower and suck him to ecstasy.

86.   Put his favorite nude photograph in his wallet.

87. Straddle him and make love in the tub.

88. Play with his male identity under the table at restaurants.

89. Buy him a sex toy and ask him to do the most creative thing he can with it.

90. Write him an erotic letter and place it in his briefcase.

91. Buy pornographic magazines and read them on long romantic drives.

92. Buy a vibrator as a gift for him.

93. Purchase sexy underwear for him.

94. Take him to a dirty movie or a live strip show.

95. Create a strip show for him.

96. Meet him for lunch in undies and an overcoat.

97. Have sex in someone else's bedroom.

98. Read him a pornographic story in which he is the star.

99. Give him a massage with oils that are sure to turn him on.

100. Have a full day of naked extravaganza: sex, photos, and more sex.

101. Suck both of his testicles, playing with his private parts gently.

102. Masturbate each other and see who will climax first.

103. Lick every part of his naked body.

104. Masturbate him in the back seat of a car.

105. Give him oral sex in the back seat of a car.

106. Give oral sex in an elevator of a tall building in any city.

107. The next time he is not interested in sex, persuade him by doing oral things to him.

108. Tie him to the bedposts and have erotic fun with him.

109. Submit to his fantasies.

110. Go without panties to the next social function and allow him to put his finger into the vagina each chance he gets.

111. Bite his nipples during lovemaking.

112. Spell out the alphabet on his male identity with the tip of the tongue and ask him to figure out the direction of each letter as it is spelled.

113. Blindfold him and ask him to guess the flavors on the vagina. Use different flavors.

114. Make love in front of a lit fireplace.

115. Make love in a taxi on the way to a favorite destination.

116. Lick the roof of his mouth while kissing.

117. Suck his male identity while he's talking on the telephone.

118. Hold his male identity while he pees, trying to guide the flow.

119. Give him a vagina massage: slowly rub it all over his body.

120. Get naked and sit on his face.

121. Lie in the middle of the table while naked and yell, "Dinner is served."

122. Tell him about her love for his hard male identity.

123. Play strip domino. Every time there's a ten-point score, remove an item of clothing.

124. Have him buy a copy of *Keeping the Home Fires Burning* and read it together.

125. Submerge his male identity into a glass of bubbly champagne and lick it clean.

126. Challenge him to make mad, passionate love for at least six hours in the same night.

127. Let him watch as a microwaved cucumber is slowly inserted into the vagina.

128. Let him watch a dildo slide into the vagina.

129. Relish afternoon sex. There is a certain sexiness this time of the day after the sun has risen and before the sun has set. It brings a sensual softness to the moment.

130. Send an exotic plant with a sexy note attached.

131. Time each other and see who can make the other climax in the least amount of time.

132. Leave love notes all through the house for him to find.

133. Slip a pair of panties in his briefcase or lunch box for him to sniff at his leisure.

134. Always smell great for him. Make it a habit.

135. Keep chilled wine ready before, during, and after sex.

136. Strip from head to toe while dancing to his favorite song.

137. Masturbate while watching him.

138. Play "find the cherry" with him. Blindfold him, spin him around, and when he finds her he gets to play with her vagina in the most sensuous and delicate way he wants.

139. Take semi-nude pictures and give them to him.

140. Suck his toes after a foot massage.

141. Lick his eyelids during lovemaking.

142. Suck his earlobes often.

143. While waiting in line together, tell him in a low, sexy voice what sexy things are going to happen when he gets home.

144. Have a mold of his male identity made for a keepsake.

145. Oil her breasts down with her favorite oils and then give him a playful breast massage.

146. Suck his bottom lip gently at the end of each kiss.

147. Become a real woman and remain one during sex.

148. Tell him that how much of a woman she is and mean it during sex.

149. Treat him like a real man.

150. Suck his fingers for no reason at all.

151. Lick his ears and his eyelids for no reason at all.

152. Have him wear a condom before every sexual encounter.

153. Go without panties all day long. It's a good way to express her sensual freedom. Slip into her sexiest underwear and ask her man to sit down. Sit astride him and then began

shaving him. Make sure to have all the necessary equipment (warm water scissors, clippers, towels). Taking care of him is sensuous and intoxicating.

Real intimacy depends on truth
—lovingly told—
especially in the bedroom.

-Joyce Brothers

Chapter 21

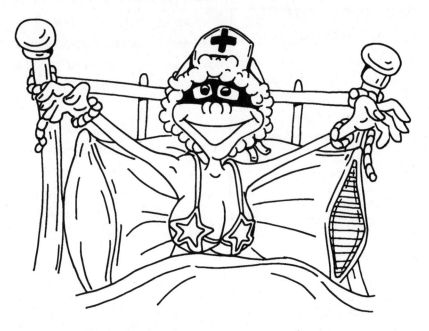

Her Places, Games, & Fantasies

Her sexual setting can actually enhance her senses.

What more could add to a woman's sexual amusement? What else can she purchase? Sexy games from sex shops, lingerie stores, catalogs, and the internet. She can create intimacy to share with her lover. The best games are those that encourage communication, arousal, and pleasure. Erotic games and fun places to explore her eroticism can add another element of fun to her sex life. One of the things most women enjoy about sexual games is the fact they do not have to limit the fun to the bedroom. A woman does not have to do it face-to-face. She can do it over the phone or email her sexual thoughts to her lover. She can text messages or play games alone. Games can happen immediately before or after sex.

Below are some fun places to have sensual moments. Her bedroom is probably the main location, but are there other places she can enjoy sensual moments that make her body pulsate at the thought of them?

> **Watch Out**
>
> Couples should create a sexual sex code. It could be as simple as, "Come find me," or "You have something in the bedroom." Making up a few sexy code words that can be texted throughout the day can be beneficial for a sensual relationship.

SEXUAL SETTINGS AND LOCATIONS

If she really thinks about it, changing sexual settings can add tremendous positive effects to the visual parts of her sexual experiences. Her sexual setting can actually enhance her senses. A couple can have sensuous moments in every room of their house or experiment with the excitement or fear of getting caught when doing it in a different place each time…maybe even public places. It is up to the woman—whatever makes her tick. Where would she have sex if she could choose? To help her with this question, here are some fun-to-have-sex locations that women enjoy. (Note: I do not condone illegal acts of sex, nor do I encourage illegal sexual activity.) A woman could have sex…

1. Under a private waterfall.

2. In the bathroom of an airplane high in the sky.

3. In a best friend's bedroom.

4. In a tree house.

5. In a chicken coop on a farm.

6. In the back seat of his or her car.

7. In an empty room next to a room full of people.

8. In the front yard at midnight.

9. In the backyard under a full moon.

10. In an empty swimming pool.

11. In a pool filled with water.

12. In the ocean at a Club Med spa.

13. In a parking garage at a Four Diamond Hotel.

14. In the back seat of someone else's car.

15. In the back of a pickup truck.

16. In the trunk of a car (make sure it has a safety latch that opens from the inside).

17. In the middle of a field of flowers.

18. On a roller coaster high in the air.

19. On top of a bar or pool table.

20. On top of a car inside the garage of her home.

21. In a secluded area of her front yard.

22. On a hidden staircase.

23. On a cruise ship.

24. On top of a printer while the butt is being copied.

25. On top of a washing machine.

26. At the ninth hole of a favorite a golf course.

27. Beneath a bridge where there is a running creek.

28. Beneath a high-rise bed.

29. Behind an extra-large, very expensive painting.

30. Behind an open door.

31. Behind a car in a full parking lot.

32. Behind a tall building, in the alleyway.

Every woman should ensure that she and her partner go on a romantically sensuous date at least once a month. Each time, they should make it a game to find a new place to have fun sex. Fun, out-of-the-way places to have sex should be on every woman's "fun to-do list."

FUN AND SPICY SEX GAMES

Here are several erotic games that will spice things up. These games and others can be found online (see "Resources" in the back of this book):

1. 365 days of romance: The sexual hope chest is useful for this one. A woman should fill it with surprising, adventurous, seductive, scratch-and-reveal cards that suggest lovemaking ideas.

2. 365 days of naughty things to do: These naughty games should be erotic and sensuous, and should be used with suggestive ideas and sex toys that are more naughty than nice.

3. Sex suit: She finds a deck of cards and picks a suit—diamonds, hearts, spades, or clubs. She and he take turns selecting one card from the deck and when pulls a suit that matches, either he or she gets to ask a sexual question or request a sexual favor. This is fun if played in the spirit of sexual exploration.

4. Sexual aim: She draws a circle or a bull's-eye on the part of his body that is a target, using flavored body paint to draw a sensuous piece of art. Afterwards, she gets thirty seconds to creatively and sensuously clear the body paint. Each player gets three chances before moving to deeper sex.

5. Do or dice: She finds some dice or square wooden blocks found in arts and crafts shops, and writes one word that symbolizes erotic or sexual instructions on each square on the blocks. Examples are lick, tickle, stroke, pump, chew, suck, bite, play, penetrate, tickle, and so on. On the other side, she draws sexual pictures, such as breasts, penis, vagina, neck, ears, and so on. They take turns rolling the dice and follow the instructions.

6. Find the position: She gets a book with lots of sexual positions and makes copies of the positions. She then folds the pieces of paper and places them in a bowl, box, or big bag. Each day she draws a piece of paper from the container and declares it the sexual position of the day. She then brings what she has chosen to the bedroom and practices. Enjoy!

7. Keep a sexual calendar: Each week, she circles a day or days in advance that are declared as her day(s) for good sex. The only rule is she must follow through on the selected date. It is especially exciting for women who are very busy or dealing with long-distance relationships.

8. Sexual fantasies: Some of the most popular female fantasies are those that are intimate and pleasurable, and arouse sexual desire. Warm feelings can come from romance, pleasure, love, and moments of laughter. Fantasy allows women to turn moments of great sex into moments of mind-blowing, whirlwind sex.

9. Sex with a lover: She imagines doing something with a lover that's more erotic and different than what normally happens with him. She can shock and surprise him with new and wonderful sex games. The choices are numerous.

10. Sex with a woman: This a common fantasy for women. Fantasizing about another woman does not mean she is into gay sex. If she loves other women, it's not abnormal to fantasize

about having sex with a woman. If she really thinks she would like this, go ahead and explore it with another willing woman. Giving herself permission to enjoy fantasies helps a woman find out what she really likes or dislikes.

11. Sex with multiple lovers: The idea of having sex with more than one person, whether male or female, is another popular female fantasy. The only reason most women don't act on it is because they are afraid of what people will think. Remember, this fantasy can bring on more headaches than needed. Sexually transmitted diseases are very common in this kind of relationship. This is not the smartest sexual fantasy.

12. Sex in a different location: Location, location, location. She can have sex anywhere she wants for as long as she wants, but please not in front of children. She takes care to make it more romantic, alluring, and sexy. She and her lover can take turns choosing a place to make mad love.

13. Oral sex: Women just love it, especially when it's done right! Enough said.

14. Forced sex: Better known as "control fantasies." I do not know many people who are into this one, but some women love the idea of being forced to have sex with their lovers. Rape fantasies do not necessarily involve trauma, abuse, or actual rape. It usually involves a rushed, aggressive need to fulfill a sexual want. Tearing clothes off, kissing aggressively, and wildly falling on the floor can bring heightened pleasure. Forced sex is wonderful when it's with the person she loves.

15. Forbidden sex: Participating in sexual acts that others feel are deviant or forbidden can turn a nice girl into a naughty little thing. Forbidden sex is the safe way to experience something

sexual that she would never really do. It's considered fantasy sex because she doesn't have to actually do it.

16. Domination: Controlling a man is attractive to many women. The feeling of power turns them on, especially power over men. They like to tell a man what to do and when to do it. They like tying him up and making him beg for love. This turns him on also.

17. Sex with a celebrity: She should imagine a favorite celebrity who can have any woman in the world, but he wants her and no one else. As he walks up to the stage and accepts his award, he thanks her for being his lover, and now the whole world knows that they belong to one another. What a fantasy!

18. Romance novels: When she is reading a romance novel, this is a chance to enjoy fantasies. She should focus on the fantasy— write it down and then act on it when he gets home. She uses sensuous terms to tell the story and gets detailed when describing sexual experiences. She can write an erotic story with her as the star, remembering to give it a happy ending.

A FINAL NOTE

This list is only a few of the ways women can satisfy their sexual fantasies. A woman should set aside other people's judgment, concerns, and comments, and let her mind go freely and get rid of all the fears. Fantasy is very important in enhancing a couple's love life. They should use the senses, create fantasies, and have fun in life and in sex.

Love is not a feeling; it's a state of MIND!

Chapter 22

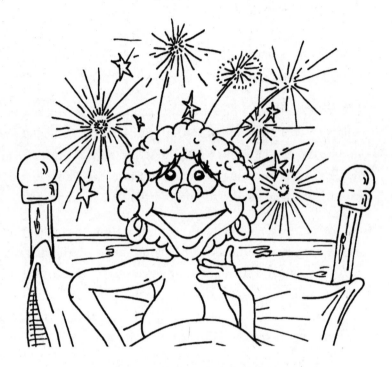

Her Orgasms

*Nearly all men can climax without difficulty,
but women just are not built that way.*

Orgasms are pleasurable and unique experiences for every woman. For
a few wonderful seconds, women can let go, lose control, and enter
a different state of consciousness. It's wonderful and heavenly. Some
women who are able to experience orgasms are becoming more and

more concerned with achieving multiple orgasms. They do not want just any orgasm. They want great orgasms. They want mind-blowing, prolonged, multiple orgasms. If it is not perfect, the woman can feel unfulfilled and disappointed.

An orgasm is wonderful, but if a woman focuses too hard on getting it, she can lose sight of pleasure. Sometime the lack of orgasm is attributed to poor vaginal health. Additionally, each orgasm can vary in overall intensity, duration, number of involuntary rhythmic contractions, and so forth. Getting serious about enjoying more sexual pleasure and achieving intense orgasms can magnify the sensations of sex. This can improve vaginal health and can guarantee amazing sex. Sex is about pleasing, giving, receiving, and sharing pleasure. Take away the pressure to achieve the perfect orgasm and she can allow her mind and body to bask in the pleasure of it all.

ORGASM FACTS

Experience of an orgasm may vary from one encounter to the next for the same woman, and even though every woman can have great orgasms, not every woman does. If a woman has either a vaginal orgasm or love button orgasm she will know it. Nearly all men can climax without difficulty, but women are not built that way. For a man sexual intercourse alone—that is, penetration of a woman's vagina by a man's male identity—may be sufficient to climax, but that's still not enough to make a woman reach orgasm. Coming is not easy for all women!

WHAT IS AN ORGASM?

What is an orgasm? Physically, an orgasm is a series of rhythmic contractions of the uterus, lower vagina, and pelvic floor muscles, which lead to a release of sexual tension. Some women have orgasms that are centered in the pelvis, while others may experience mental imagery or auras. Orgasm is the pinnacle of sexual passion. It is that moment of intense pleasure, which results in feeling relaxed and at ease. The female orgasm lasts a few seconds, followed by a feeling of relaxation and pleasure. Continued stimulation may also result in further orgasms.

TYPES OF ORGASMS

There are two types of orgasms women experience, based on the two different zones of stimulation. The first is a love button orgasm, where light touching, massaging, or stroking stimulates the love button. The second type of orgasm is a vaginal orgasm. This comes from pressure being applied to the G-spot (see "Stimulating Her G-Spot" in Chapter 14), usually by the tip of the man's male identity.

Both experiences are very different, and women who have experienced both kinds of orgasms know the difference. Few women reach orgasm solely as a result of the male identity (penis) penetrating the vagina; it's likely to happen through stimulation (touching/rubbing/kissing) of the love button, the highly sensitive bump located at the top and in between the vagina lips.

FACTORS RESPONSIBLE FOR ORGASM

- Sexual frequency. In order to reach climax, it is important that a woman has regular sex. The more time that passes between sexual encounters, the harder it is for her to become aroused and the less likely it is for her to have an orgasm.

- Relaxed and tension-free environment. For a woman to get the most out of her sexual encounters, she must be comfortable with the relationship and the situations she is involved in. Orgasms are impossible in situations where there is tension or lack of trust. She must relax and release.

- Understanding, caring, and attentiveness. A person's lover should be someone who knows how to stimulate and arouse and who helps her reach a climax.

HOW MEN HELP WOMEN REACH ORGASM

For a woman to reach orgasm, it is very important for the man to co-operate with her and understand her and her body. She should not be so shy that she cannot tell him how to make love to her and what arouses her. Knowing which part of her body will make her climax is helpful to the both of them. When a woman makes love, she should guide the man, helping him help her reach orgasm. Here are some important things that will help the woman become relaxed.

- ❦ The man tells her she is marvelous, sexy, and beautiful, and means it.

- ❦ He stimulates her love button by gently massaging it.

- ❦ He makes sure to touch/kiss/stroke in succession, which will help her reach wonderful orgasms.

- ❦ He performs oral sex on her if she wants. Some women adore oral sex and claim they cannot come unless a man "goes down" on them.

- ❦ He caresses her breasts and gives attention to her sensitive spots. Few women climax through breast fondling alone or by stroking their sensitive spots, but it sure does help.

- ❦ A man should ask the woman to show him what she wants.

- ❦ If the man comes before the woman, he should try to help her climax by kissing and stimulating her continuously.

- ❦ He should always help her feel safe. He should try his very best to provide an atmosphere of love, romance, security, and compassion.

WAYS SHE CAN TREAT HERSELF

A woman who experiences no or few orgasms can learn to bring herself to climax with patience and self-stimulation. It takes time to learn the sensitive spots and the best touches, interpret feelings, and understand thoughts that arouse to the point of climax. These techniques are practiced alone and then later with him. A woman should:

- Avoid trying too hard. Focusing on the orgasm risks increasing anxiety and short-circuiting pleasure and orgasmic responses. Relax and focus on the emotional, spiritual, and physical pleasures of lovemaking.

- Explore her body. When alone, she can touch and stoke it in ways she would like to be caressed by her lover. Learn to enjoy those things that really stimulate her.

- Share her experiences. Once she knows what stimulates her to reach climax, she communicates these things to her lover. Guide him to parts of the body that are aroused when stimulated, and then she can find other pleasurable ways to arouse herself too.

- Let him stimulate the love button during foreplay, until she finds herself on the brink of orgasm.

- Move into intercourse. After her lover has touched and caressed her love button, he moves straight into intercourse, remembering to stimulate her love button.

- Add toys to her pleasuring moments. Try the Hitachi Magic Wand. The intense vibrations are sure to help her along the way. It can help increase the number of orgasms she achieves (see "Battery-Operated Boyfriends" in Chapter 24).

- Practice Kegel exercises every day (see Part 4, "Stimulating Pleasures"). Exercising the pelvic floor muscles makes the vaginal muscles strong and increases blood flow. Orgasms are more intense when the pelvic muscles are stronger.

- Be patient. Sex improves over time. The more comfortable and relaxed she is, the better the sex.

- Release and let go. Practice breathing in a relaxed state. Accept the pleasure. She deserves it.

ORGASMIC STATES

Some philosophies have two ideas about orgasm: the physical orgasm and the heart orgasm. At first appearance, they may seem dualistic and contrary, but on closer inspection, one supports the other perfectly.

The orgasmic state of "being," which is considered the bliss-state,

> **She Should Know**
>
> She should get fired up! Prior to sex, she could take a hot bath or place a warm washcloth over her vulva for a few minutes. Heat boosts blood flow to the vagina, leading to increased lubrication and sensitivity.

is associated with the energy transferred to all that we are and do during the day. On the other hand, however, sexuality itself is used to reach the deepest spiritual levels a woman can attain. The orgasm is the gateway to recognize this bliss-state. Modern women recognize that there are several forms of orgasm. Let us discuss them.

1. Love button (clitoral) orgasms tend to be more localized to the genitals. The vagina orgasm mostly involves the G-spot and a few other locations in the vagina. As implied, love button orgasms come from direct stimulation of the love button and surrounding area. Most women only experience love button orgasms.

2. Blended orgasms involve both the love button and the G-spot, as the love button splits into two roots under the skin, wrapping around either side of the G-spot and stimulating it directly.

3. Energy orgasms, or heart orgasms, are a result of superior sexual health. If a woman has good sexual health, she will experience amazing, frequent, and intense energy orgasms.

4. Full-body orgasms lend themselves to full-body orgasmic potential when the breath, the mind, and the orgasm itself come together. With this full-blown experience with different breath patterns, sounds, and techniques, a woman has the

potential to move into multiple orgasms and out-of-body sex. Going even further into this practice, she is able to have full-body orgasms, or energy orgasms, simply by breathing deeply with small amounts of physical touch.

5. Vaginal orgasms, including G-spot orgasms, occur during intercourse or by direct stimulation of the G-spot. It is often described as deeper and more intense than love button orgasms. Many women have never had a vaginal orgasm. Just as with a love button orgasm, if she has good sexual health, she will experience bliss.

6. Multiple orgasms are deliciously unforgettable. This is the ability to have repeated orgasms within a short period, e.g., a single lovemaking session. In order to achieve multiple orgasms during intercourse, good vagina health is essential!

7. Ejaculatory orgasms are known as natural occurrences for some women and are coupled with incredibly intense orgasmic pleasure. There is one constant with women who experience ejaculatory orgasms: they have great sexual health.

SOME ORGASMS ARE DIFFICULT TO ACHIEVE

Sometimes a woman will not be able to experience orgasms, no matter how hard she tries. Here are some possible reasons an orgasm might be difficult to achieve.

- Fear of not having an orgasm.
- Physical factors. One example of a physical factor negatively affecting orgasm is fatigue. If her body and mind are tired and need rest, an orgasm is unlikely.
- Fixation on orgasm. She thinks too much about whether she will have an orgasm and not about how aroused she is or isn't.

❦ Overthinking things. She wonders what her lover thinks of her. These concerns make it difficult to climax. Instead of focusing on the sensations of the sexual encounter, she is thinking about all the could of, would of, and should of's.

❦ Length of time since last orgasm. In order to reach climax, it's important that she has regular sex. The more time that passes between sexual encounters, the harder it is to become aroused, and the less likely she is to have an orgasm.

❦ Pressure and tension. She might be afraid or ashamed of asking her lover to arouse her, and as a result, she ends up being unsatisfied. In addition, she is afraid that if her lover concentrates on her pleasure only, she'll feel pressured to do the same for him, which leaves her incapacitated sexually.

❦ Rushing into sex. Not leaving enough time to get fully aroused to climax results in the orgasm getting pushed aside during sex.

❦ Psychosocial factors. These include her mood, relationship to her lover, activity before sex, expectations, and feelings about the overall experience.

❦ Feelings of guilt. Family, religion, and moral values often shape beliefs about sex. She has always thought of sex as something dirty or something that she should not enjoy. The guilt gets in the way of her true enjoyment of the experience.

❦ Low self-confidence. Negative feelings about self will inhibit her efforts to feel good about sex. Some women are so ashamed of their bodies they are not comfortable while making love. They simply do not enjoy the thought of sex, even though they do want it.

❦ Past relationship traumas. What happened in the past can play an important role in whether or not she can relax enough to make love. When a woman is traumatized, enjoying the entire sexual experience can be difficult.

THINGS THAT HELP ACHIEVE ORGASMS

There are ways to achieve satisfying orgasms that women will love. Most important, a woman must relax and focus completely on the sexual act. To open the door to sexual satisfaction and pleasure, a woman should:

- Resolve conflict. Communication between partners is very important when finding out what stimulates and turns a woman on. If she has a problem, she must speak up. The two should talk about all facets of the relationship with one another. Unresolved conflicts can put the damper on sex and orgasm.

- Let go of inhibitions. Fear, embarrassment, shyness, and mental blocks are all factors that keep a woman from having an orgasm. She keeps her mind clear and enjoys sex instead of depriving herself of pleasure.

- Get to know her body. She has to be sufficiently aroused to reach orgasm, but to get sufficiently aroused, she needs to know what makes her feel good. To start, she should set aside twenty minutes of uninterrupted time. While taking a relaxing bath, she looks at her naked body in a mirror. After looking at her body, she closes her eyes for a while and quietly examines the mental picture of her body. Once comfortable, she puts some lubricant on the finger and touch the vagina lips, love button (clitoris), and inside the vagina, finding out which areas are most sensitive and what touch feels good.

- Self-touch in ways that heighten arousal to the point of orgasm. Where does it feel better? A woman should know more about her body than the man does.

❦ Try new positions. Trying new positions helps her achieve different kinds of orgasms. To achieve an orgasm with G-spot, she needs stimulation. So, she should try a position that will stimulate this spot, leading to an orgasm. Experimenting with many positions, she will find the ones most likely to lead to orgasm.

A SENSUAL NOTE

For some women, difficulty in experiencing orgasm is the result of physical problems, chemical or hormonal imbalance, drug or medical side effects, or even previous psychological trauma. Such situations may require more extensive sex therapy or treatment. To better understand problems, she should discuss them with a doctor or therapist.

If he was like any of his music, he would be complex, explosive, sweet, sensual, and passionate.

~Kailin Gow, The Protege

PART 5

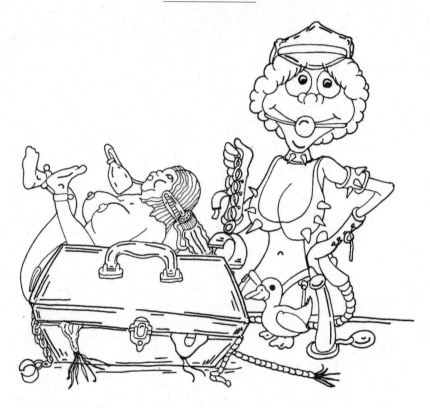

Pleasure Containers, Prop
Boxes, Hope Chests & Supplies

Chapter 23

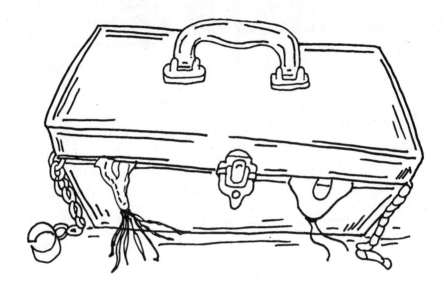

Her Pleasure Containers

A woman will need more than one place for all her props and supplies.

Sexually active women should have containers they refer to as their sexual hope chests, pleasure bags, or goodie drawers. Pleasure containers hold sexual toys, props, and supplies. They are made from a variety of small, decorative cardboard boxes, straw baskets, and plastic or metal containers. A woman's pleasure container could even be an extra drawer that is used for nothing except sexual supplies and toys. This container or drawer should safely store, hide, and preserve her sex toys, lovemaking props, or sensual supplies, and should consist of items that add variety and spice to her sexual experiences.

Exploring the use of sexual props and supplies does not mean a woman will not be able to have heated passionate experiences without them. She should think of sexual accessories in the same way a framed picture on the wall adds to the beauty of the room or a piece of jewelry or a scarf adds to a wardrobe. Using sex toys, games, and accessories adds spice and excitement to lovemaking. Every woman should have some sort of sexual accessory.

HER PROP BOXES AND HOPE CHESTS

Listed below are sensuous items that can fill her pleasure container. Whether she names it a goodie bag, prop box, or sexual hope chest, there is probably something in her home she can use to make one. She should try some of the following supplies and have fun with them.

1. Whipped cream is inviting and used on all parts of the erogenous zones. Some favorite places are nipples, stomach, navel, neck, ears, toes, buttocks, male identity, fingers, and any other hot spots. But she should be careful not to get it inside the ears.

2. Assorted lingerie is nice to wear at any time. Men admit that a woman in beautiful lingerie is a turn-on. She can watch the sparks fly when she unveils her body dressed in beautiful attire. She should make sure that bras and panties match, and are fresh and sexy when sharing time together. It adds flavor to the mood.

3. Sunglasses in assorted styles with beautiful frames are glamorous when worn correctly. When wearing casual clothing, casual sunglasses are appropriate. When wearing glamorous attire, she should wear a pair of glasses that will fit the occasion. Every woman should have more than one pair of sunglasses in her wardrobe.

4. Men's suits are hot on a sensuous woman. Wearing a man's suit adds flair and helps the man to chill out. Sensuous suits turn men on. She should pair the suit with a low-cut blouse or no blouse at all, and accessorize with small, delicate jewelry and sexy underwear.

5. Nail polish adds allure and beauty to a woman's nails. Clear polish is sensuous on clean, manicured hands. Color can send sexy messages to men.

6. Fruits like bananas, strawberries, cherries, and pineapples are nice additives to oral sex. If she likes to have sex and eat it too, she should try tasting pieces of fruit before, during, and after sex.

7. Long coats are nice when visiting him—wearing nothing underneath except underwear. She should wear a long coat over nice lingerie in his favorite color. These long coats can be thought of as long dresses.

8. Oils and lotions are enriching to the skin when available for a nice massage before or after sex. Men love sensuous massages at any time.

9. Toiletries are great when a lover sleeps over. Having a few items in his favorite brand is considerate and in tune with his needs. She should keep a little container or basket under the counter for him with toothpaste, colognes, shaver/razor, comb, brush, after-shave, and so forth. Having the things he needs will make him feel more connected. In addition, he should do the same for her.

10. Aprons are great for sensuously greeting him at the door. By wearing nothing but an apron tied around her sensuous waist, she can watch his excitement grow.

11. Popsicles are a terrific turn-on as he watches her use them to penetrate, lick, and penetrate again. Used as erotic foreplay, this works wonders. Assorted popsicles are good too.

12. Chilled wine or champagne is stimulating when poured over his body and licked off. Champagne is used for dipping pleasures, so she should dip his male identity into a glass of champagne and lick it off. It will give him goose bumps and turn him on. He will immediately rise to new heights.

13. Mr. Goodbars are given as a sexual gesture to tell him he's good. The best time to send him a Mr. Goodbar is the day after sex. Send it to him wrapped in gift paper or in a gift box by a delivery company. He will ring her phone off the hook after he receives it.

14. Breath mints are a handy necessity for any woman who kisses and talks to someone up close and personal.

15. Having fresh condoms is not only smart, it is also wise. Smart and sensuously mature women are responsible for their own sexual protection. Condoms have a shelf life, so she must make sure the condoms are not old and outdated by checking the expiration date on the package. This influences the effectiveness of protection. She should also use spermicidal jelly with condoms—twice the protection is great.

16. Incense, potpourri, or other aromas set the mood and enhance the atmosphere. Aromas create waves of erotic moods. It helps her think sexy thoughts.

17. Candles are romantic, soothing, and alluring when used with her lover. When she is alone, candles add a special and personal atmosphere. They lull her to moments of subtle interludes. It is

pleasant to watch television, take a bath, or just sit and talk by candlelight. Who can resist being romantic when the setting is so mellow?

18. Lights and illuminations are nice peeking in from other rooms. Dimly lit or colored lights add romantic overtures and decrease electric bills. The magic of subtle lighting is enchanting.

19. A tape measure comes in handy for measurement games with her lover. If he is confident about his sensuous area, it is fun to measure the length and width of it. But she must not use this as a ridicule tool. It should only be used to get a rise out of his male identity.

20. Costumes are a nice turn-on for men. A woman can keep him at home by changing how she looks for his pleasure. Men like the idea of having more than one woman. So why not make herself into that multiple person? She can change her hair, clothes, and any other features from time to time to add spice to an otherwise routine relationship. She might dress up to look like his favorite starlet or sex goddess, or create a look for him. He will be surprised at the efforts to please him.

21. Handkerchiefs squirted with a little perfume are nice to carry in her bra, purse, or pocket. It makes for a beautiful scent on her body.

22. Love notes are great messengers. She should leave them everywhere he will be. Keeping them simple and personalized, she should be sure to say little things in notes that push his erotic buttons. If she jots down something that only he can relate to, he will understand the message being sent.

23. She can create scenes by decorating the home or apartment for a romantic trip. If her favorite place is Rome, she can do as the Romans do and invent pleasures from the scenery to the food. Her objective is to create a wonderful and romantic

atmosphere of love for two. She can stop by a travel agency and pick up brochures and travel information, and then add little props like souvenirs. The key is for them to escape entirely by playing the role completely.

24. Sweet additions like syrups, jellies, honey, sugar, chocolate, and other delights can add tasty pleasures to her appetite. Especially when she uses slow, seductive licks to eat it off him. She alternates tongue motions by slipping and sliding the tongue in continuous lavishing licks. This one will send chills throughout his entire body, and his excitement will in turn arouse her.

25. Balloons or flowers are fantastic when trying to make up or add cheer. Balloons can be kept in the prop box, or she can send balloons or flowers and a message to let him know that she is thinking of him. He will be shy, but the idea will send happiness to his brain.

26. Picnics can be in the park, living room, back yard, on a patio, or even in a bedroom. Fireplace picnics are a favorite also. She should simply prepare a picnic basket with a favorite wine, cheese, and foods, and select a place to enjoy it. The two of them should indulge in the fun of it all. Maybe a nude picnic at home? She should try it and not forget to add sensuous and spicy ideas.

27. Pearls are nice when worn alone. She greets him at the door wearing a single strand of pearls, and if he can guess how many pearls are on the strand, he gets to choose his sexual pleasure for the day.

28. Silk scarves should touch him lightly all over his naked body. She can use silk scarves as halters, aprons, and veils, or maybe even a G-string before stripping in front of him to music.

29. *Keeping the Home Fires Burning* is the theme of the night.
    Recite the parts that turn him on, and if he gets turned on
    before she finishes, simply make love—don't worry.

A SENSUAL NOTE

A woman will need more than one pleasure box or sexual hope
chest for all of her props and supplies. One box is for sexual items,
and another is for those things that are edible. Yet another one is used
for things she has to replace or clean on a regular basis, such as tooth-
brushes, soaps, lotions, and so forth. Whatever she decides, she is sure
to keep them clean, handy, out of sight, and away from children. She
should not forget to add special props or accessories to this list.

Every woman should have her own props and supplies on hand,
in addition to ordinary sex.

Chapter 24

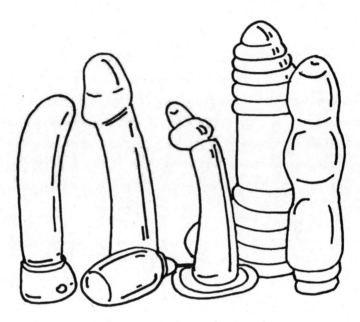

Her Sex Toys, Props & Supplies

*When deciding to look at a variety of toys, a woman should think about what
is sexually compatible.*

Every woman should own a few sex toys for private pleasure and sex
play. Owning a few sensuous toys can help her gain a better understanding of her body and heighten her overall sexual experience. While
the majority of sensuous toys look like male identities in different sizes

and colors, there is a wide variation available. Sensuous toys that penetrate the vagina are available for all size preferences, from extra thick and stubby to long and slender.

Some are smooth and featureless, while some have detailed veins and family jewels. Some stimulate the G-spot or prostate and have undulations, bumps, angles, or corkscrews for extra sensation.

When a woman wants a tune-up or an extended sensual session, her battery-operated boyfriends (BOBs), known as vibrators, are the ideal sex toys to get her motor revving and send her racing to a 400-horsepower orgasm. Battery-operated boyfriends come in a phenomenal array of types and sizes.

Using battery-operated boy friends is great if a woman wants to learn her own sexual likes and dislikes. Vibrators are among the most widely used and available toys, and because they come in such a variety of sizes, shapes, colors, and materials, they are great for vaginal, clitoral, or anal

> **Watch Out**
>
> Not washing her toy, using the wrong lube, or storing it incorrectly can lead to problems—from a shorter lifespan or distortion of a toy to the risk of infection for her.

stimulation, and can be used internally, externally, or both.

Some vibrators serve as body massagers, relieving more than sexual tension. There are vibrators that work by battery, and there are those that plug into the nearest electrical socket. There is even a model that can plug into the car's cigarette lighter.

HER BATTERY-OPERATED BOYFRIENDS/ VIBRATORS/DEVICES

There are also special battery-operated boyfriends, battery-operated toys, and/or battery-operated devices. Each is designed to fit perfectly between a woman's legs, around the head of a guy's male identity, or neatly in anyone's anus. The BOB can produce a soothing sexual feeling or an intense one, depending on how one uses the gadget and how one is sexually wired. Those adventurers who want their orgasms to be more portable will find a huge variety of battery-operated vibrators that start to look more "penile." There are vibrators that look nothing at all like a male identity. Those that are not-so-male-looking are easier to travel with.

Thanks to recent developments in the kind of plastic used in vibrators, they are more lifelike, feel both incredibly realistic and hot, and are more than a little creepy. There is even a new series of realistic vaginas available (with or without vibration), so those who prefer to make love rather than be made loved to can share in new state-of-the-art technologies.

One thing that's great about modern sex toys is that while it's possible to make a toy that looks like a penis or vagina, added special features will also stimulate a love button or other private parts.

Some of these pleasure toys look like totem poles with the head of a polar bear attached (the bear's tongue working the love button), or the head of a dolphin (with the dolphin licking at the little man in the boat, aka clitoris).

Finding the best model may take a little self-lovemaking research. When deciding to look at a variety of toys, a woman should think about what is sexually compatible and ask herself a few questions:

1. "Do I like penetration, love button stimulation, or both?" "Do I find it more stimulating when my partner plays with my love button, penetrates my vagina, or both?" The answers will help

determine which type of vibrator is best. Some vibrators are made for external use only to stimulate the clitoris, others are designed to enter the vagina, and some can stimulate both at the same time.

2. "Will I need lots of power or more intensity?" All vibrators offer something different. Before buying one, she should consider the intensity of the vibration that will bring pleasure. An electronic vibrator produces strong vibrations and will not run out of energy as quickly as a battery-powered device, and may be worth its weight in gold if used for long periods. The best way to find what is best is to visit a retailer that has a multitude of different models.

3. "What toys are aesthetically pleasing to me?" "What is the attraction of the toy?" If she does not like the way a vibrator looks, it is going to be very difficult to get comfortable using it. A woman who wants to be more discreet can find something as unassuming as a tube of lipstick.

4. "What do I like or dislike?" Using a battery-operated boyfriend is great for a woman to learn her sexual likes and dislikes. Using them with relaxing music and an erotic atmosphere makes the mood perfect.

It is important for her to relax and breathe deeply. She should concentrate, use the battery-operated boyfriend in different positions, and receive different degrees of stimulation. She uses it until just before climax, takes it away, relaxes, and begins again. Using the battery-operated boyfriend allows her to achieve multiple orgasms and learn how to enjoy sexuality. Men are not the only ones who can masturbate.

Keeping battery-operated boyfriends clean is the ultimate way to practice safe sex. All that's needed is knowledge about using them. If the vibrator is not waterproof, she doesn't put it in water. A vibrator is designed to stimulate and bring pleasure. It does a better job of stimulating than a tongue, finger, or any inanimate object. It is a perfect masturbation tool for both women and men, and can greatly heighten sexual intensity for women. A woman should do what feels good with it. There is a definite difference between battery-operated boyfriend orgasms and orgasms produced by other means. A BOB orgasm is more intense, and it's common for women to have multiple orgasms while using it. Consistent and intense stimulation of the love button is normally required for a woman to climax. The BOB is great at that.

WHAT SEX TOYS ARE MADE OF

Garden-variety sensuous toys are made of rubber and/or vinyl, but high-quality toys are made of silicone. They are nice, firm, and a little more expensive. They feel good, and silicone is more durable and easier to clean than other materials. They require careful handling but are worth it for the realistic sensations.

When visiting a sex shop, a woman should notice what the sensuous toys are made of. From plastic and rubber to glass and steel, selecting the perfect toy can be a dilemma. She must consider comfort; how realistic it will be, how pleasurable it is, and how easy it will be to take care of. Here's an easy guide to help:

- Cyberskin feels and looks like the real thing and is not very high maintenance. Toys made of this material are very porous and difficult to clean, and get a little sticky after using. To maintain the soft skin-like feel, it helps to cover them with a small amount of cornstarch before storing them. Bacteria and yeast can get trapped in the toys and may cause chronic vaginal infections. The best bet is to use condoms on vibrators or dildos made of jelly rubber or Cyberskin, which needs replacing more often than toys made of other materials. Again, a woman should always cover the toys with a condom to keep them sanitary and bacteria free.

❧ Glass is also used for dildos, a type that is great for G-spot stimulation. Glass dildos can be warmed and chilled for different sensations, and the nonporous material is easy to clean. Most are marketed as shatterproof, but care is needed, because rough handling can break them. Glass toys are often hand blown and quite beautiful. Displayed on the coffee table, they will not be recognized as sex toys. Glass toys are cleaned with hypoallergenic soap and water.

❧ Plastic is nonporous, hard, durable, and easy to clean. In the past, plastic toys used to be simple hard plastic, but they broke, developed stains, or cracked when used. Now, however, there are materials available that are so lifelike and comfortable that a woman would be hard-pressed to tell if it was a live male identity or a gadget. Warming plastic toys with water before using them gives a more realistic feel. Plastic is the best material for intense vibrations but tends to be a little louder than other materials. Plastic toys are cleaned with soap and water.

❧ Jelly and rubber toys could get picked out of a lineup and easily compare with real male identities. Jelly vibrators provide a variety of fun. Often coming (pun intended) in vibrant colors, their "skin" is soft and jiggly, like a sort of aroused cup of Jell-O. One bit of advice when using jellies is to keep them in a plastic bag and try not to let them fall to the floor, as they have a tendency to collect lint and dirt. Otherwise, they are truly fun to play with. Jelly rubber is a porous rubber blend that has a soft feel that many women like, and it holds its vibrations better than rubber latex. Unfortunately, it is difficult to clean since over time lubricants and body fluids get trapped in the pores and create stickiness. It should be cleaned with soap and water and replaced after a few months of use.

❦ Steel can also be warmed or heated and is nonporous, so it's easy to clean. However, the feel is far from realistic.

❦ Silicone is the most popular material for sex toys, perhaps because it warms up to the body's temperature, maintains heat, and is easy to clean. If it is waterproof, it can be boiled for three minutes to sterilize it or cleaned in the dishwasher. Toys made of silicone can last a long time. I do not recommend using silicone-based lubricants on any silicone toys because they can damage them.

HER TOP BATTERY-OPERATED TOYS

These toys are sexy, guaranteeing hours and hours of wild orgasmic fun. There are other, sometimes even more surreal, devices as well. Additionally, there are specially ringed vibrators just for men, as well as toys for women called panty vibrators (wearable vibrators). First, let's take a look at a few toys.

1. The Pocket Rocket is a small rocket-shaped vibrator that looks like a little pocket torch in appearance. If a woman purchases only one toy, this is my recommendation. The Pocket Rocket is a tiny but powerful "massager" that is only about four inches long. It can fit in a small purse, and it looks like a tube of lipstick. It transforms when placed in a jelly rubber sleeve. It comes in delicious colors, such as blueberry, grape, lime,

strawberry, and tangerine. Jelly rubber sleeves shaped like a bunny (with extra-long ears) or a variety of other textures can be added. Lubricating this one yields wonderful pleasure.

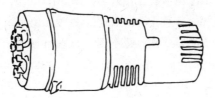

2. The Hitachi Magic Wand is still the Bentley of vibrators. It is a large electronic vibrator that is just as effective for relaxing tired, sore back muscles. as it is great for producing intense orgasms. It's sold in the small appliance section of many department stores, as well as in adult sex shops. This enormous, two-speed plug-in model possesses a sturdy wand handle and a huge vibrating head. What is new about it is that there are now attachments fitting onto the head that focus on love button stimulation. The Hitachi Magic Wand is the most popular version, but other comparable handheld models are available.

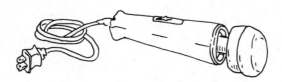

3. Jack Rabbit is a more elaborate creation. It is sold under several brand names, but the name rabbit was made more popular by the *Sex and the City* cable television show. It features multiple elements and moving parts. They do every-thing except sing. This dual vibrator is the ultimate sex toy. It is not recommended for beginners. Most feature a rotating chamber of beads, or "pearls," in the shaft, which tumble against each other, creating extra movement and sensations

inside the vagina. At the base of the shaft is
a cute rabbit, beaver, or dolphin that buzzes
and bumps against the love button. Deluxe
models feature a rotating male identity. Some
come with an anal tickler. All these elements
have separate controls and varying speeds.
This is one of the only vibrators that stimulate
several areas of the vulva and the vagina at the
same time. It runs on four AA batteries. The
combinations boggle the mind, not to mention
the coochie. These models cost a bit more and are
generally well-made and worth it for an ultimate
vibrator experience.

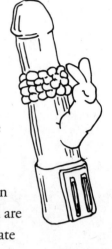

4. Dildos are basic penis-shaped toys, which are
    used to practice fellatio and perfect the hand
    job. A dildo is used alone or with a partner
    to stroke the cervix or penetrate the vagina.
    Dildos are cast from molds of real penises
    complete with veins and testicles.

5. G-spot Vibrator is easy to detect due to the
    curve at the top of the shaft. The curve allows
    the top of the vibrator to press against the
    G-spot when inserted in the vagina. There is
    also the G-spot Vibrator dildo without the vibrations.

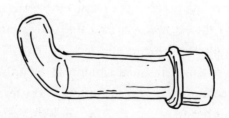

6. Finger Vibrator is the perfect way to introduce toys to a male partner. It is placed on his finger, allowing him or her to maintain control. It is less threatening for the man who has fears that toys will replace him. The vibrations are perfect for stimulating the vulva and love button. It is used to simulate his penis or perineum too.

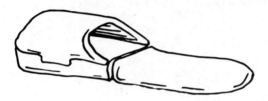

7. Natural Contours Vibrator looks more like a small medical device than a sex toy. It is sleek, smooth, and designed to fit along the natural curve of the vulva. The vibrations are gentle and comfortable. It is perfect for the woman who is new to sex toys, as well as for the more experienced woman.

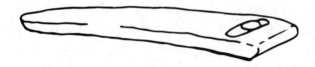

8. Vibrating Bullet is a tiny powerhouse and is capable of creating pleasurable sensations for both partners. It's made to stimulate the clitoris and fits on top of or between the outer labia. A woman simply drops the bullet into her panties and sits back to enjoy a private party. The bullet is also great for partnered sex. Place it against the love button while having intercourse for erotic pleasure.

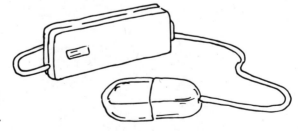

9. Strap-on Vibrator makes it easier for women to reach climax during intercourse. The straps hold it in place against the clitoris while leaving the vagina and anus free for intercourse. It provides additional stimulation for ultimate pleasure.

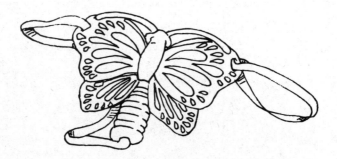

10. Cock Rings, as the name suggests, are rings that fit over the penis shaft, encircling the base of the penis, or the penis and the testicles. Cock rings restrict blood flow out of the penis, which keeps it engorged and helps the erection last longer. Rings may be made of plastic, rubber, leather, or metal. One word of caution: blood flow out of the male identity should not be restricted for an extended period (no more than twenty minutes). A man should choose rings that are adjusted with snaps or made of stretchy rubber so they can be removed easily (and quickly in case of an emergency). Stay alert: the ring should not be used if it is too tight or causes pain.

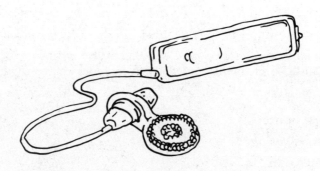

11. Vibrating Cock Ring is a stretchable cock ring that is placed at the base of the erect male identity. The attached vibrating egg should be rotated at the top of the ring, so when a woman has intercourse, the vibrating egg has contact with her love button, providing additional stimulation during intercourse. The man can feel the vibrations at the base of his penis and scrotum. To increase clitoral stimulation, the woman assumes the woman-on-top position and grinds her hips against the egg attachment.

12. Butt plugs are designed and worn for the feeling of fullness. They are essentially small dildos designed to fit and stay in the anus. They have a flared bottom that prevents them from sliding too far up the rectum. They are made of silicone or rubber and are easier to use than they sound. They are also easy to clean. Some butt plugs come with heart-shaped bases, and the silicone is excellent for conveying vibrations—all she has to do is put a vibrator to the base. The plugs come in a variety of shapes and sizes. There is the long, thin, pointed plug; the shorter, flatter, slightly curved version; and the small, squat, fat-beaded version. Plugs that are more than four inches long should never be used, as they could cause internal damage.

13. Flex-O-Pleaser has a small battery pack, a long neck, and a vigorous head—just the thing to get to the small of her back, or his prostrate or G-spot, for that matter.

14. Ecsta-Sleeve Vulva is a stretchable sleeve made of Cyberskin that fits over the male identity. It includes a vibrating egg for stimulating the sensitive head of the male identity.

15. Ball Collar attaches around the man's family jewels, and he can add weights to it. Men love this kind of pressure.

16. Neptune Ring Valve is a tiny vibrating dolphin attached to a male identity ring. This works either by giving her lover a solo buzz or by stimulating the love button during intercourse.

17. Gummy Bear Ring is a jelly rubber male identity attachment that fixes at the base of the male identity (or dildo). The blue model comes with a mini-probe for focusing on the G-spot, and the red model comes with little side flaps that tickle the love button.

18. Raspberry Ring is a raspberry-shaped stimulator fitted to the front of the ring and is said to be the most effective shape for love button stimulation. The ring is made of aqua blue silicone.

19. Sensa-Touch Wand by Dr. Scholl's. Dr. Scholl has graduated from sandals and is now selling his own version of the Magic Wand.

20. Attachments. What is special about the last two vibrators is that there are some cute pink or purple G-spot attachments than can also be used to give the prostate a massage. Plus one has a slender, curved tip specially shaped to give maximum pressure on the front wall of the vagina, where the infamous G-spot is located. The latest models do more than vibrate. They pulsate, which may be integral to a woman's style of orgasm, especially for G-spot stimulation. They are a lot quieter and can be turned on without everyone knowing.

21. Pulsatron has several different speeds. It throbs and pulsates. The user can choose the speed with the touch of a switch.

22. iSurge Vibe has several variations, which include vibration, pulsation, escalation, and roller coaster.

23. Spiral Plug comes in metallic black and includes a removable tiny vibe. It nestles perfectly into its base; it is a quiet and reliable vibrator made of good-quality silicone and is excellent for prostate or vagina sensation. It requires three watch batteries (included) and has one strong speed.

24. Rub My Duckie looks like a rubber duckie, and it floats like a rubber duckie, but when squeezed, it buzzes and vibrates. It's the ultimate vibrator disguise. The beak and tail stimulate the love button.

25. Bottoms Up Kit includes a book titled *Anal Pleasure and Health* by Jack Morin, which is considered the bible of anal stimulation. Also included is a lavender jelly rubber Arrow Twist Vibrator, which probes and promotes thrilling interior sensations. It comes with batteries and a bottle of special lube.

26. Fukuoku is a small, quiet vibrator designed to fit neatly over the end of a finger, basically turning the woman's finger into a tiny vibrator. The Fukuoku can reach all those hidden areas and a few obvious ones too.

27. Fukuoku Gloves are also available, making each fingertip into an epicenter of tiny tremors.

28. Fukuoku 9000 is one of the newest vibrators. Working off tiny watch batteries, it fits over the finger like a tiny finger sheath and vibrates. There is no battery pack and no cord. It's perfect for surprises during intercourse, since it is virtually undetectable. The kit includes textured rubber pads to fit over the device so that it can vary finger sensation.

29. Thai Beads are a string of three small pearly-pink beads to be inserted into the anus and then pulled out slowly. They are used to accentuate stimulation or in a rush for a great climax.

30. Jumbo Beads are a graduated, larger version of Thai beads.

31. Jelly Beads, often referred to as jell beads, are spongy, ruby-colored, equally sized jelly beads with a ring pull that offers a firm, jelly-like sensation.

32. Double Delight is a hands-free, two-ended BOB that is supposed to be worn by heterosexuals when the man enjoys anal penetration.

33. Mini-Hummer vibrators offer targeted vibration for women who find it difficult to climax. It is strapped into place over the love button, held on by an elastic waist strap and leg straps. It is great during sex because it hits the right spots.

34. Triple Stimulation is a male identity ring with a flexible dildo for penetration of the anus while the vagina is penetrated.

35. Bullet Vibes are small vibrators encased in an egg- or bullet-shaped capsule and are popular because of their compactness and the punch for their size. They are used directly on the love button, inserted in the vagina, or combined with other toys. Many BOBs, butt plugs, and male identity rings are designed to be infused with a jolt of juice. The vibe is attached via a small cord to a handheld battery pack/controller.

36. Wireless versions are also available, but users must be careful not to lose track of them in an orifice. Other very small vibes run off watch batteries, which are enclosed in their case. These little battery-operated toys may look too small to be more than a novelty, but they really do work.

JOY BUZZERS

These are on-the-go vibrators that are small, hidden, and fun to own. They are great when a woman has to sneak away to have self-pleasuring time.

1. Vibrating Panties are underwear with a mini-vibe tucked inside and can be worn without detection under regular garments. She should get one with a remote-control unit to add spice to a night on the town.

2. Butterfly, Scorpion, and Dragonfly are wearable units that feature probes and plugs combined with a small vibe to tickle the love button, vagina, and butt. Tiny clip-on vibes are clamped to the nipples, love button, or labia for intense sensations.

3. Tongue-Joy is for those who like to give more than receive. The mini-vibe that straps onto the tongue gives a little oomph to oral sex. Put on a single finger, it becomes an instrument of exquisite pleasure.

4. Buzzing Buddies vibrators are not just for the ladies. Vibrating jelly male identity rings slide over his male identity and sit snugly at the base. They usually feature nubs or probes that contact his lover's love button during intercourse. For a real hummer, he can put a vibe under his ball sack, against his perineum (the spot between his family jewels and anus).

5. Strap It On. For no-hands with a lover, a strap-on dildo works well. These strap-ons are suitable for use by women, as well as men who want to enhance or maintain an erection.

6. Ride That Dong. To make love and really grind on that male identity, she can get a dildo with a suction cup base that can attach to the wall, shower tiles, floor, or other smooth surface. Some women stabilize dildos by bracing the base with pillows.

7. Get a Buzz. A vibrating dildo or multifunction vibrating dildo can provide extra stimulation along with penetration. These vibrators can also be used externally on the vulva, love button, or male identity and testicles for masturbation.

TOYS FOR MEN

Male sexual pleasures have many layers. The reason that anal stimulation is such a hot topic is because men have a G-spot too, and the anus is the access point to the male G-spot. There are stunning sensuous wands designed for both external and internal use. Learning more about a man's sexual anatomy and his varied range of pleasure zones will expand lovemaking to different kinds of arousal and enjoyable sensations. Interestingly, some of the same deep, intense internal orgasms that women find when locating their G-spots are also available for men.

She Should Know

Silicone: She should wash with soap and water or place it in the top rack of the dishwasher. She can also put it in boiling water for ten minutes to disinfect.
Glass: She can wash with soap and water, but it should not be exposed to extreme temperatures.
Pyrex: It is heat-resistant glass, so it can be boiled, put in the dishwasher, or washed by hand.
Stainless steel: Boil for ten minutes, soak in bleach and water, and then rinse thoroughly.

Working with prostate massagers and identifying how to locate and stimulate the erogenous area require trust from both partners. The nerve endings between the anus and the scrotum are a surprise for men, but they react better when a gentle and patient hand is used in the beginning.

A toy that every woman should add to her intimacy resources is the C-ring, also sometimes referred to as P-ring or erection ring. Most have vibrators attached, and some have a double-ring system to fit around the base of the penis and wrap around the scrotum. These toys help men maintain an erection because when they use the ring, the blood flow is caught in the erect penis and the scrotum. The vibrating part of the ring is turned to face behind the scrotum, stimulating the nerve of the perineum toward the woman, which directly stimulates the clitoris during penetration. Regardless of the location of the vibrating element, the sensation of the penis vibrating inside the vaginal cavity adds a completely new dimension to lovemaking.

Luxury versions of multiuse toys are rechargeable. The medical-grade silicone stretches to fit any size and is softer and suppler than the single-use models. Just like their female vibrators, they recharge like a cell phone. It is used with or without the vibrating attachment. For all penis rings, the standard safety recommendations suggest use for no longer than thirty minutes at a time. Some men have difficulty ejaculating with them on, so removal prior to orgasm makes sense. For other men, orgasm is easy and more exciting with the ring in place.

> **She Should Know**
>
> Some porous toys can't be completely disinfected, so she should always use a condom when using it with a partner. If she's using the toy on herself, she should be fine as long as it's washed after every use.

TOYS THAT PLUG IN

Toys that women like plug in too. The classic BOB is battery powered, phallic shaped, and made of plastic, silicone, or a similar material. It is stroked, inserted, or held against the genitals. The most basic of these is the standard smooth plastic vibe. These were once sold in the back of magazines as "facial massagers." They come in a dazzling rainbow of candy colors, neon, and glow-in-the-dark and light-up models. These are not average massagers, and women should never believe they are! They pack a punch for sexual satisfaction throughout the sexual activity and gratification being the end result.

Other insertables incorporate the vibrator into a realistic dong made of rubber, jelly-rubber, vinyl, or silicone. With so many sizes, colors, and styles available, there has to be one that will appeal.

> ### She Should Know
>
> She should remove batteries from the toys when they are not being used. Leaving batteries in can corrode the toy and drain battery life, since they're conducting at a low charge when in the toy. There's nothing sadder than the halfhearted buzz of a vibrator with spilled battery acid or on low batteries.

AVOIDING TOY DAMAGE

A tiny nick on the surface of a jelly rubber, silicone, or Cyber-skin dildo can turn into a big tear that will ruin the toy. Care must be taken to keep the dildo away from sharp or pointy objects or abrasive surfaces, and its life can be prolonged by storing in a box or protective cloth or bag when not in use. Less common are "Swedish" type massagers that are strapped onto the back of her hand, thereby turning her whole palm and fingers into a vibrator/massager. These produce a very intense vibration that some find wonderful and others find overwhelming.

SECURITY CHECKS AND BATTERY-OPERATED BOYFRIENDS

Everyone has heard horror stories about someone getting pulled out of the airport screening line because there was a vibrator hopping around in their luggage. There is a simple way to avoid this embarrassment: remove the batteries before packing. For discretion, one should consider getting a vibrator that is not shaped like a male identity or the standard vibrator. There are many nonphallic vibes designed to fit the shape of a woman's vagina, resembling a high-tech electric shaver instead of a sex toy. Others are shaped vaguely like flashlights, while some are disguised as rubber duckies or small dolls. Mini or finger-sized vibes are also a good choice because they easily slip into a pocket or purse.

BATTERY-OPERATED BOYFRIEND TIPS

To get maximum pleasure from a vibrator, as well as to prolong the life of the device, a woman can:

- ❦ Experiment with positioning to get the best sensations. Going straight for the sensitive areas may not work best. Vary pressures and, if the vibrator permits, try changing the speeds.

- ❦ Try using the vibe on the outside of clothing or through layers if it is too intense.

- ❦ Watch out for "vibrator dependency." Vibes will not deaden a woman's sensations, but she may get used to them and find it difficult to come with other stimulation.

- ❦ Lube can reduce friction and intensify sensation, whether inserting the vibe or just stroking the sensuous spot.

- ❦ Test the vibe on other body parts (e.g., thighs, buttocks, breasts). Those sensuous ripples of pleasure are great.

- ❦ If she is planning to use the vibe in the bath, be sure to get a waterproof model. *Do not use electrical vibrators near water.*

- ❦ Clean the battery-operated boyfriend regularly with soap and water, or according to its manufacturer's directions.

- ❦ Remove the batteries during cleaning and do not get water in the battery compartment. It will rust the inside metal parts.

THE DOUBLE DILDO IS A VERSATILE SEX TOY

The double dildo is one of the more exotic sex toys. A standard prop in girl-on-girl activity, it is actually a versatile toy for either gender, or for individuals in solo masturbation. Here is a rundown of the many ways to use it:

1. A double dildo is designed for two people to be penetrated simultaneously, but it can also be used for solo masturbation.

2. Vagina to vagina: Two or more women use a double dong for simultaneous vagina penetration. A man and a woman can use it to find more pleasures that stimulate his prostate and her G-spot.

3. Vagina to butt: The female is penetrated in her vagina while her lover takes the other end of the dildo in the butt.

4. Butt to butt: Two lovers of either sex can use a double dildo for simultaneous anal penetration.

5. Double penetration: If the dong is flexible enough, a woman can insert one end in her vagina and the other in her anus for double penetration.

6. Solo masturbation: A double dong is used like a regular dildo.

7. Penetration during masturbation: The user grips the free end as a sort of "handle."

A woman can use her creative juices to come up with many more possibilities. Has she ever wanted to suck the male identity and eat vagina at the same time? Have her insert a double dildo and then go down.

1. Face-to-face: The lovers lean back and insert the dong. Best for vagina to vagina.

2. Side by side: The two lie side by side, prop one leg up slightly and insert the dildo. Lie face-to-face for vagina-to-vagina sex.

3. Vagina to butt: The lover receiving the dildo anally should lie with their back to the other.

4. Back to back: Both lovers kneel on all fours facing in opposite directions. They back up toward each other as they insert the dildo. Works best for butt to butt, but can also work for vagina to vagina or vagina to butt.

Getting started is easiest if one person inserts the dildo first, and the other moves toward them and inserts the other end. The act is a little tricky, as it is easy for the dildo to slip out while pumping on it. During sex, one person may have to hold the dildo in place to keep it steady. Although two people can bang away on opposite ends of a dong, it works best

> ### She Should Know
>
> She should look for signs that it's time to throw the toy away. Even the best toys don't last forever. If the motor gets louder, it's a sign that the toy is getting to the end of the charge. If the charge isn't lasting as long, that could mean it's no longer nonporous. RIP.

if one lover remains more or less stationary. One person can grip their end of the dong and grind into the other person, or they can hold it in place while the other person rides their end. One of the great things about a double dong is that it is an equalizer, and both can take turns being active and passive.

HER BEHIND

A few cautionary words are necessary concerning the use of double dongs for anal penetration. If one end of a double dong is used in the anus, that same end should never go into a vagina without being thoroughly cleaned first. Inserting an object in the vagina after it has been in the butt spreads germs that can cause yeast and internal bacterial infections. For safe and pleasurable use of a double dong, both parties should:

- As with any sex toy, take precautions when sharing so no infections or STDs are transmitted. Do not insert a dildo into one person and then insert it into another without cleaning it between lovers. Be sure to clean the toys thoroughly after use, or cover them with condoms before use for easy clean up.

- ❦ Be sure not to push it so far into the butt that the whole thing slides up and gets stuck. It is best to insert toys in the butt that have a flared base, like butt plugs, to keep them from slipping in past the anal sphincter.

- ❦ Get the right model. Most double dongs are long enough to keep a grip on the free end, and users are not likely to lose the whole thing. However, if the hands are slick with lube and it is pushed a little too far, a woman may find herself stuck in a very embarrassing predicament. If concerned about the double dong getting lost, get a model with a flange or family jewels in the middle that will stop it before it goes too far. Scary but true.

OTHER DOUBLES

If the double dong is not her style, or she is looking for something more ergonometric for dual penetration, a woman could try a strap-on with a vagina plug in the harness. The harness holds the smaller dildo inside.

Other double dildos, such as the Feeldoe, the Nexus, the Boomerang, and the Super Penetrix, are V-shaped dildos designed to have one end held in place by the wearer's vagina muscles. The other end of the dildo sticks up out of her crotch at an angle like an erection, allowing the woman to make love as if she were wearing a strap-on.

The vagina dildo is usually a bit larger and thicker, while the anal dildo is smaller and curved to meet the inner contours of the body. These toys are suitable for masturbation rather than with a lover. To use the double dong, one or both parties should:

- ❦ Use a water-based lube, like K-Y Jelly or Astroglide, to make insertion easier. Water-based lubes are compatible with all sex toy materials and clean up easily.

❦ Start with one end. Let one lover get the dong inserted before the other tries to get their end in. Trying to get both ends inserted at the same time will result in the dong slipping around too much.

❦ Take turns with him. Double dongs are great equalizers for heterosexual women because both partners get to make love at the same time. Take turns being the active or passive lover. One partner can hold the dong in place inside her and make love to the other with it.

❦ Double her pleasure with double penetration. A woman can insert one end of a flexible double dong in her vagina and one end in her butt. This works best with dongs made of jelly rubber that are sixteen inches or longer. Insert one end and hold it in place, and then push the free head into the other hole.

❦ Use the free end. While masturbating with a double dong, rub the other end on her love button, or give it a hand job. There is a whole other male identity sticking out there, so put it to work.

❦ Grip the end to use the double dong as a make love tool. Use one end of a double dong for the same purpose. The nonlubricated free end of makes a convenient "handle" for loving herself or a friend.

❦ Use separate ends of the dildo for anal and vagina insertion. If using one end of a double dong anally, be sure not to use that end for vagina insertion until it has been thoroughly cleaned.

SEX TOY WARNINGS

For safe use of sex toys, a woman should:

❦ Avoid using oil or petroleum-based lubricants (like Vaseline or Crisco) if the male identity toy is made of rubber or Cyberskin; instead use a water-based lube (like Astroglide). Greasy stuff will cause rubber male identities or BOBs to disintegrate.

❦ Prevent the toys from getting lost. If using a rubber toy for anal pleasure, be sure it has a flared base big enough to keep it from disappearing up the butt.

❦ Resist letting the eyes be bigger than her, um, orifice. To get an idea of how much she can comfortably handle, test-drive a clean cucumber or zucchini. Whittle it if needed until she gets the right proportions, and then measure the length and circumference. Put a condom on the vegetable for added protection against infections. Remember that pesticides are used on fruit and vegetables. Imagine explaining a pesticide infection in the vaginal area to a doctor. Clean the vegetables well.

❦ Guard against germs. If sharing the toys with a lover or using it in more than one orifice (e.g., the vagina and the anus/butt), either clean the dildo thoroughly between insertions or use condoms on it and change them between insertions to avoid STDs or germs that cause infections.

❦ Always keep it clean. Clean sex toys after every use by washing with mild antibacterial soap and hot water, or use a disinfectant sex toy cleanser. Sticky dildos can breed germs and attract dust and dirt that can cause serious infections.

A SENSUAL NOTE

A woman should be careful about inserting one of those slick plastic numbers. If there is nothing at the base to keep it from slipping up inside her, it will be embarrassing if an ER doctor has to extract a still-buzzing sex toy from the body cavity.

Whether she is after a quickie or an extended sensual session,
vibrators are the ideal sex toys to get her motor revving.

Chapter 25

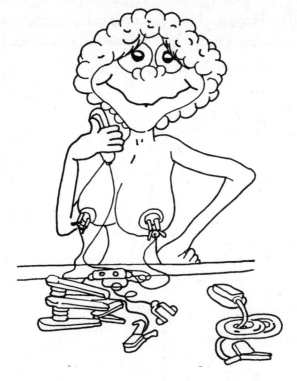

Her Sensuous Clamps

*The main purpose of nipple clamps is not to inflict pain, but to provide
constant, intense nipple stimulation and heightened sensitivity.*

Women-owned-and-operated sex businesses have made it their mission
to take sex toys out of the dark and into the light. If men think sex toys
are just for them, they can think again. They are not! There is a whole

new unbiased world for the sexually interested female, and she has many kinds of sex toys to choose from.

It seems that women have always possessed hungry orifices, and there are many new sensuous toys that have been added to the list of toys that probe (and vibrate). There are those that gently constrict and amplify (male identity rings), those that imitate (false vaginas, plastic tits), and those that restrict (bondage implements). Yet, for the most part, sex toys buzz or are inserted wherever it feels good.

Most any woman can find a reason to use sensuous clamps. They add excitement to lovemaking. They are used in addition to the sexual hope chests, props, and supplies. Most adventurous low-key toys are included in the clamp category. They might consist of: (a) handcuffs, in black leather and fluffy trimmings, (b) self-adhesive tattoos, (c) PVC blindfold (kinky heart-shaped bottom paddle), (d) fur collars and leads, and (e) nipple chains.

There are two kinds of clamps: the wand and the coil. Wands are powerful and have many speeds, like large plastic flashlights with a vibrating head at one end. The coil type usually has a much higher vibrating rate and is smaller, with a pistol grip. Neither of these types of toy looks like something a woman would clench between her thighs, but she should not let that dissuade her from giving them a try.

Giving and Receiving

Rubber tips are perfect for newbies and the easy-to-use sliding ring allows for pleasure control.

BUZZING CLAMPS

There are some special buzzing devices that come with gentle and not-so-gentle clamps. These are tiny vibrators that work directly on the nipples and are fed by a small controller and battery pack. In their simplest form, nipple clamps are a variation of an alligator clamp with an adjustable spring or locking device. Each of the clamps is attached to a chain in such a way that pulling on it tightens the grip. The tip is covered with a cork, soft vinyl, or rubber, both for traction and to give some cushioning to protect the skin and tissues.

- ❦ Forceps designs are great if she is into doctor/nurse fantasy or medical fetishes. They look like a pair of scissors and have a locking device between the arms to hold them in place.

- ❦ Tweezer clamps are just miniature tweezers or tongs encircled by a metal band that slides upward to tighten them. Their ends are covered with rubber or vinyl cushions.

- ❦ Clover clamps resemble a pair of pliers with two round, flat pads that compress the nipples.

NIPPLE CLAMPS

Nipple clamps have a chain that keeps the clamps together as a set. The chain adds a little weight and gives women something to tug on to manipulate the clamps. Sexually submissive types get excited at the thought of being led around by the tits.

Nipple clamps are ranked highest among the bestselling devices. Despite their name and appearance, nipple clamps are not torture devices. They have a reputation as sadomasochism toys, but women don't have to be into heavy kink to enjoy them.

The main purpose of nipple clamps is not to inflict pain, but to provide constant, intense nipple stimulation and heightened sensitivity. They actually squeeze the nerve endings. Both men and women get some level of erotic response from having their nipples squeezed, played with, bitten, or sucked.

> **She Should Know**
>
> If she isn't ready for or isn't interested in metal clamps on her nipples, but still wants to explore nipple play, she should try the silicone nipple suckers. They give a similar feel with less pressure.

Nipple clamps provide stimulus while freeing a woman's hands and mouth to do other things. They put constant pressure on the nipples, which is intensified with added weights, vibrators, or manual tugging. This heightens the nipples' sensitivity during play.

NIPPLE JEWELRY

This kind of jewelry combines form and function. These trinkets are mostly for women and are worn by women on their nipples, but men like them too. One type is a sort of lock with a springy, open, metal circle with covered ends that tweak then close the nipple between them. Tension from the end that simulates a lock holds it in place, and the effect is like a nipple ring without the piercing.

- Elastic loop or adjustable lasso goes around the nipple, often with beads, feathers, or tassels attached.

- Weights and vibrators are other add-ons that heighten the effect by pulling on the nipple. They swing as she moves.

- Deluxe nipple clamps come with mini-vibrators attached for really over-the-top stimulation and are a great multipurpose toy as well. The clamp is used on the love button and family jewels, and is clipped either directly onto those body parts or on underwear so that they nestle against the private body parts.

If a woman has a pierced nipple, she should remove any jewelry before attaching the clamp or position it perpendicular to the piercing. Because piercing can stimulate growth of nerve endings in the nipples, increasing sensitivity, she may need to use less pressure with the clamps.

NIPPLE CLAMP APPLICATION

Nipple clamps are applied with care. To get them properly adjusted and placed, a woman should:

W Put the clamps on slowly and tighten carefully. If the nipple clamp has a screw adjustment, tighten it slowly until she achieves a pressure that will hold the clamp in place without causing too much pain. If the clamp has a simple spring mechanism, place the open clamp around the nipple and release slowly, so pressure is applied steadily to the nipple. Do not let it snap shut.

W Tough it out. The initial pressure of the clamp may feel intense and may even be slightly painful for the first couple of minutes. But the pain will gradually dull and give way to a warm throbbing and tingling, especially if she is already aroused. At this point, she may find that her nipples are hypersensitive, so that the slightest brush or tug on the clamps produces overwhelming sensations. With vibrating nipple clamps, she will want to wait until she reaches this stage before turning the vibrators on.

W Restrict their use. Nipple clamps compress delicate tissue and restrict blood flow. They should not be worn for more than fifteen minutes at a time.

W Know when to stop. Discontinue use and remove the clamps if she experiences real pain (as opposed to pleasurable pain), if the skin becomes broken, or if the nipple turns blue or purple. If she does sustain a nipple bruise or injury, ice it to reduce swelling and discoloration.

W Use caution. For some people, nipple clamps are part of a more involved nipple play scene, which may involve nipple bondage (tying ropes or cords around the breast or nipple) and pumping (using suction pumps or snakebite kits to pump up and enlarge the nipples). Please read all directions on the clamps before use.

W Be aware of long-term effects. If she uses nipple clamps occasionally, it is unlikely she will experience any permanent changes in her nipples as a result. However, frequent tweaking may cause slight enlargement of the nipples and prolonged heightened sensitivity.

❦ Adjust pressure during period. A woman's nipple sensitivity varies during her menstrual cycle. Adjust the pressure of the clamps as desired.

❦ Go undercover. Vibrating nipple clamps are nice on the love button or family jewels. Attach to the inside of undergarments for an undercover buzz.

❦ Remove carefully. When the clamps are removed, hold steady so that they do not hurt when taking them off. Removing them can actually be more painful than putting them on, because the sudden rush of blood circulation back into nipple brings back feeling to the area. The nipples will be extremely sensitive for a while. Try having her lover blow on them or brush them lightly with his lips or a feather and see what happens. Later, massage gently with some lotion or have her lover help ease the sting.

WARNING ABOUT TOYS FOR PREGNANT WOMEN

Pregnant women should use caution when engaging in clamped nipple play. Stimulation of the nipples releases the hormone oxytocin, which causes uterine contractions and may induce early labor in the later stages of pregnancy.

To love oneself is the beginning of a life-long romance.

~ Oscar Wilde

Chapter 26

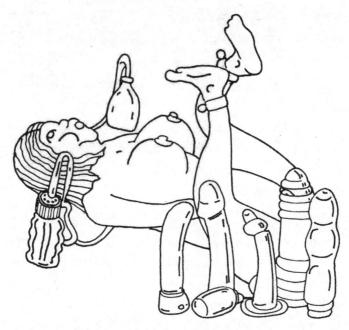

Her Cyberskin Toys

"Sex is a natural function. You can't make it happen,
but you can teach people to let it happen."

~ William Masters

Toys made of Cyberskin and similar soft, flesh-like materials go by various names: Softskin, Ultraskin, Futurotic, and so on. They are made from a high-tech rubbery polymer, or thermal plastic, whose silky texture and pliable consistency are amazingly lifelike. Unlike regular rubber or silicone, Cyberskin does not feel cold to the touch, and it quickly warms to body temperature. It's very stretchy, soft, and flexible, which makes it an ideal material for a wide range of sex toys.

- Cyberskin dildos are among the most realistic penis-like toys available, not just for their appearance, but also for their skin-like surface and soft-yet-firm density.

- Some Cyberskin male identities are so detailed that they have skin that moves along the shaft and family jewels that shift inside the scrotum. If a woman wants a dildo that feels like the next best thing to a real male identity, Cyberskin is the way to go. And if she wants to use it with a friend, she should get a Cyberskin double dong.

- The skin-like texture of a Cyberskin male identity makes it a pleasure not only to make love to, but also to suck and touch. But Cyberskin does requires special handling—care must be taken not to nick the surface of it, because it is delicate and can tear very easily. She should think of it as actual flesh and treat it with sensitivity. Because it is semiporous, it is more difficult to clean than other materials.

- It is best to cover the Cyberskin dildo with a condom before inserting it, especially if using it for anal penetration or sharing it. In addition, as with all Cyberskin toys, only water based lube should be used. Oil-based or silicone-based lubes will destroy Cyberskin material.

If she is rough on sex toys, or prefers a harder and hassle-free kind of lovemaking, she's better off with a dildo made of rubber, latex, or silicone. Cyberskin vibrators and vibrating dildos are exceptionally kind to her delicate areas. Because Cyberskin is so soft, it can absorb vibrations; a small vibrator inside a thick Cyberskin casing may produce a barely perceptible buzz. For more powerful sensations, larger vibrators with thinner Cyberskin surfaces are better.

CYBERSKIN VAGINAL STIMULATORS

Cyberskin is also a popular material for strap-on vibrators that focus directly on the love button. Elastic straps hold these small vibrators over the love button, as the Cyberskin casing stimulates the love button, labia, and vagina. Although most are too large and awkwardly shaped to wear under clothing, the soft material is comfortable against the skin.

- The lifelike properties of Cyberskin, as well as its stretchiness and pliability, make it an ideal material for vagina stimulators and masturbator sleeves. Simulated vaginas are molded to resemble the female genital area and are modeled to accept a male identity for more simulated intercourse. To be clear 'stimulators' are used to arouse and 'simulators' lean more toward molded fake vaginas.

- The Cyberskin replicates the feeling of flesh and stretches to accommodate and hug the inserted male identity. For those who are more interested in the male anatomy, there are Cyberskin male identities and anus simulators.

- Many vagina simulators come with an anal aperture as standard equipment, so couples can pick the orifice they want to stimulate.

- Male masturbator sleeves differ from realistic vaginas in their size and design. Vagina sleeves give a little more to grasp on to and are designed for simulated lovemaking. The masturbator sleeve is held in one hand and used as a sexual accessory. Sleeves may be molded in the shape of a miniature vagina or lips to simulate the man's penis head. Rather than make love to them per se, the woman inserts the male identity into the snug sleeve and strokes it up and down.

- Cyberskin masturbators may not look like much, and she may look at the tiny hole in the end and wonder how even a modest-sized male identity could get inside. Cyberskin proves to be a wonder material with an amazing ability to stretch, without tearing or losing its shape.

- She can find a male identity mold maker in her city and arrange to visit it with her lover so he can get a mold made of his male identity.

- Male identity extensions fit over the male identity to add length and girth. Cyberskin extensions have the benefits of both feeling extremely lifelike and being comfortable to wear. They come in strapless and strap-on.

- A Cyberskin extension must be handled carefully when putting it on and taking it off. It is flexible and stretchy, so rolling it on and off is as easy as taking off a condom. The person removing the extension should not tug or pull at the end or the edges.

- Most Cyberskin male identity rings are designed to fit around the base, above the family jewels. They help maintain an erection by slowing the flow of blood of the male identity.

- Cyberskin male identity rings also lend themselves well to the addition of love button–stimulating knobs or vibrators. Because it restricts blood circulation, a stretchy male identity ring must not be worn for more than half an hour.

CLEANING AND STORING CYBERSKIN TOYS

To prolong the life of her Cyberskin sex toys, a woman should:

- Wash them with warm water and mild or antibacterial hand soap after using. Pat dry with a clean cloth or paper towel.

- Do not rub Cyberskin toys roughly, as this may abrade the surface or rub lint onto it. If it's an extension, masturbator sleeve, or vagina simulator, wash and dry it inside and out.

✿ Put about a quarter cup of cornstarch into a Ziploc baggie or Tupperware-type plastic container with a lid and then drop in the Cyberskin toy. Seal the bag or container and shake thoroughly until the toy is coated. The cornstarch keeps the surface of the Cyberskin from getting sticky and prolongs its life. If it is a sleeve or extension, make sure the cornstarch gets inside as well. If the toy is too big to fit in a bag or container, apply a light coat of cornstarch with the fingers.

SENSUAL NOTE

Talcum powder or baby powder should not be used to dust Cyberskin toys. Talcum powder has been linked to cervical cancer. Even though cornstarch will cake on, when it is removed with a tissue or cloth, the Cyberskin will be smooth as a baby's bottom. The woman dusts off the toy; wraps it in a clean, dry cloth; and places it in a clean Ziploc bag for storage in a secure place until its next use.

Using sex toys is really a matter of personal preference.

Chapter 21

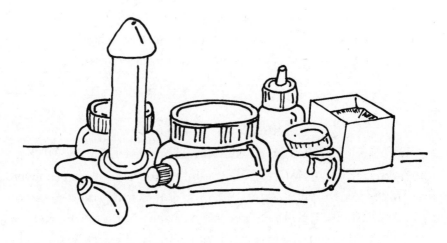

Her Lubricants, Gels, Oils, and Creams

Even though natural lubrication is the preferred fluid, it is always nice when a woman has options.

Women and men love lubricants. Even though natural lubrication is the preferred fluid, it's always nice when a woman has options. There are times when a woman's vagina becomes dry, which makes it difficult to receive easy penetration during lovemaking. Lack of lubrication is the number one reason condoms break. If a woman is looking for personal lubricants or wonderful sexual lubricants, she should look no further.

There are a wide variety of sex lubricants that help a woman slip and slide her way to safe sex.

Dry vagina is a common problem for many women who are experiencing menopausal symptoms or some kind of hormonal problem. Because of the reduced levels of estrogen, women may not secrete enough fluid to have normal lubrication, so lubricants are great sex aides.

She Should Know

Lube has the reputation for being something one pulls in off the bench during penetrative sex when a partner is having a harder time maintaining lubrication. This is total BS. Her partner should place some in his palm and gently grind her vulva and labia against it for a new twist on the hand job for women.

Lubricants such as Vaseline or baby oils can cause holes in latex condoms, so it's best not to use them. Coconut oil is a good option. The major complaints about lubes are that they have artificial ingredients, they taste bad, and they have a numbing effect. Below is a list of popular lubricants, oils, creams, or pills. Any woman who needs a lubricant can take a look; maybe she'll find one she likes.

LUBRICANTS AND GELS

1. Sensua Organics offers the world's first all-organic personal lubricant, made from whole, certified-organic, food-grade ingredients. The peach and raspberry formulas have a light, fruity scent and a mild, all-natural taste. The unflavored formula is odorless and tasteless. In addition to being the healthiest choice, Sensua Organic's innovative formulas allow for continuous rehydration by using the body's own moisture.

2. Homeopathic Luscious Flower Libido Formula. The original organic homeopathic personal lubricant is specifically designed to increase desire and sensation, while promoting a healthy response in women.

3. K-Y Jelly safely replaces personal moisture in a way that feels natural and helps enhance sexual pleasure. K-Y lubricants are condom safe, rinse off easily, and can be used every day. K-Y lubricants are thoroughly tested and proven safe to use.

4. Bliss Lube is not only natural, it also does not numb the mouth. It is a lightly vanilla-flavored liquid, is not overwhelming, has a bit of sweetness (without sugars), and does not have that chemical-soapy smell that other lubes have. It has nature's purest ingredients. It's a personal lubricant that works with the body's natural chemistry to enhance moisture and glide. This water-based formula is nonirritating and long-lasting for naturally pure pleasure. If a woman is concerned with the effects that chemical lubes might have on her body, Bliss Lube is water based, pH balanced, and made with minimal, natural ingredients without any harsh petroleum derivatives. There are also no paraben preservatives or propylene glycol. It is a bit more expensive than some lubes, but in lubes, as in life, she'll get what she pays for. Bliss Lube contains natural aloe vera, which has been known to be a natural spermicide. However, it's probably not wise to use it as a spermicide. It's one hundred100-percent natural, pH balanced, petroleum free, water based, paraben free, sweet tasting, nonstick, and latex friendly.

5. Very Private is a daily intimate moisturizer created specifically to counteract vaginal dryness. Very Private helps ease the beginning of pleasure and gives maximum tissue protection, literally cushioning the vagina tissue with moisture so sexual activity is completely comfortable and can last as long as desired. It's extremely effective and consumer friendly, and feels as natural as a woman's own moisture—no stickiness, no residue, and no superfluous ingredients to change the natural vagina environment. Thousands of women use it for

combatting vaginal dryness with great satisfaction. Very Private is also recommended by several teaching hospitals, such as the MD Anderson Cancer Center and Cedars-Sinai Medical Center departments of gynecology, and it is FDA approved to be marketed as a 501(k) medical device. It feels as natural as a woman's own fluid and adapts to her body's temperature.

6. Astroglide is a favorite that's sure to please. Astroglide is water based and water-soluble, petroleum free, light, odorless, colorless, tasteless, no staining, and long-lasting. It contains no spermicide and will not harm condoms! What more could a woman ask for in a sex lube? Astroglide is second only to nature. Astroglide now comes in a Sensual Strawberry lube, and it has been found in some studies to inhibit cell replication.

7. Venus for Women is a clean, safe, highly concentrated, moisturizing massage lubricant designed especially for women. Venus pampers the body, leaving skin velvety soft and smooth. Venus is composed of the highest-quality clinically tested ingredients. It is safe to use, nontoxic, and hypoallergenic. It is perfect for women with extra-sensitive skin. Venus is extremely long lasting and does not block pores. It contains no preservatives and it's oil, water, fragrance, and taste free. It never dries out or gets sticky. Latex safe, Venus is perfect for body massages and moisturizing.

8. Aqua Lube is from the makers of Kimono brand condoms and is specially formulated to enhance sensual pleasure by supplementing the body's own lubrication. Aqua Lube is odor free and nonstaining, and will not harm condoms. If a woman is looking for frictionless pleasure, she will love this product! Aqua Lube is available without spermicide in two convenient sizes.

9. Foreplay is a sensual water-based lubricant. It is one of the most advanced lubricants available. It is no staining and completely edible, and has a pleasant taste. It is safe to use on condoms. Foreplay is also pH balanced for sensitive skin. It comes in a nine-ounce bottle, in regular formula or enhanced with aloe vera and vitamin E.

10. ID Glide is a water-based lubricant that stays slick longer and does not gum up or get sticky. ID Glide is unflavored, no staining, and fragrance free. This product is safe to use on condoms.

11. Wet Light Lubricant is the longest-lasting, most-dependable personal lubricant available. It's colorless, greaseless, and odorless, and a favorite among lubricant lovers. It is water based, oil free, and safe to use with condoms. Wet Light is a lighter, thinner liquid version of Wet Original. Both are without spermicide.

12. ID Millennium Never Drying and Super Slick are the leaders in long-lasting lubricants. Using a special silicone-based formula, ID Millennium is latex friendly and will stay slick even underwater. Available in two-ounce and eight-ounce sizes, the advanced formula makes ID Millennium the preferred choice in high-end lubricants.

13. Eros Body Glide is a revolutionary new moisturizing lubricant from Germany, which was recently introduced into the United States. Eros will never get sticky or dry out, and it easily absorbs into her skin. One drop is all it takes. It takes less and costs less. Eros is hypoallergenic, tasteless, fragrance free, and oil free; it does not stain; and it protects the skin without blocking pores. Eros will enhance any body-to-body experience and is produced under the strictest European clinical standards and completely safe with latex.

14. Sylk is tasteless, odorless, and nongreasy. Sylk mimics the natural vagina juices and is safe to use with condoms.

15. Wet Platinum is a top-quality lubricant. It comes in a sexy black bottle and stays wetter and slipperier for longer than any lubricant tested in clinical trials. It is used by men and women, and is safe to use with condoms.

16. Spike Anal Lubricant is by Doc Johnson. It comes in a concertina-shaped squeeze bottle with long probe applicator for delivering deep inside.

17. Chocolates or homemade gelatin is great when she indulges during oral sex. The sweetness flood her lover's genitals with sweet-smelling edibles.

SEX OILS

Even when her sex life is going well, a woman can find ways to make it better. The following sex oil lubricants will add positive spice to lovemaking.

1. Zestra is plant-based oil that increases arousal, vaginal lubrication, and sexual pleasure in some women. The oil is massaged on the love button, labia, and opening of the vagina prior to sex. The effects begin five minutes after application and last up to forty-five minutes.

2. ProSensual is a soy-based lubricant that is described as a topical sexual stimulant for women. When applied to the vulva, it may increase arousal and sexual pleasure. Some women describe a warm, tingly sensation after application.

SEX CREAMS

For women who want to give their man the pleasure of a lubricant, there is the ever popular, most familiar, and most reliable of sexual pleasures—male cream. Male creams enhance the sensation and augment pleasure to satisfy a man's personal and sensual needs.

1. Forever Hers is a prolonging emollient. It makes pleasurable moments last. This amazing cream temporarily desensitizes and will increase any man's staying power for prolonged sexual pleasure. Mild yet cool and fresh, Forever Hers is vitamin E enriched, water soluble, condom safe, and made from pure food ingredients. It comes in a two-ounce jar. There are two flavors to choose from, crème de menthe and passion fruit.

2. Durex Maintain Sex Lubricant for the man who desires a little extra staying power. It is a desensitizing lubricant to prolong sexual pleasure for both lovers. Maintain is water based, clear, odorless, and safe to use on condoms. A little dab on his male identity and he'll stand at attention all night. It comes in a one-ounce tube.

3. Viacreme offers women enhanced physical sensation. It is safe and natural and made just for women!

4. Vivid Virility is an fast-acting supplement that creates longer, stronger, harder erections within minutes! Vivid heightens sexual drive and desire as a man's male identity engorges with increased blood flow.

Because reduced levels of estrogen in women may cause a lack of secretion or limit normal lubrication, lubricants are great sex aides.

SENSUAL NOTE

There are many other lubricants available. For great finds check out:
http://www.annsummers.com
http://www.goodvibes.com

> *Sensual and spiritual are not easy words to use*
> *that there are perhaps not two*
> *Aphrodites but one Aphrodite with a Janus face.*

> ~E.M. Forster, The Longest Journey

Chapter 28

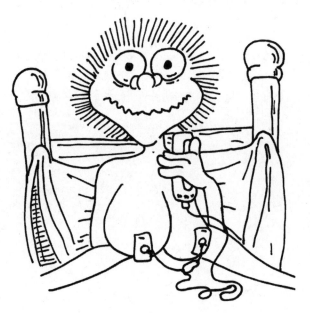

Her Electricity

"She worked her toes into the sand, feeling the tiny delicious pain of the friction of tiny chips of silicon against the tender flesh between her toes. That's life, like electricity. It hurts, it's dirty, and it feels very, very good."

– Orson Scott Card

There is always the kind of emotional intensity that sparks electricity between two lovers. There is also the kind of electricity that's used to excite lovers with safe, low-voltage mini-bolts of electricity. It's the infamous TENS unit machine, a small, box-like piece of equipment used in physiotherapy to send small electrical charges into the skin to relieve physical pain.

The electricity I am speaking about in this chapter is for the enhancement of sexual pleasure. It comes in minimal doses and, unbelievably, women who use it really like it. They give it their stamp of approval. To be honest I have never tried it, but I couldn't resist including it in this book. The lengths people will go to find and get pleasure fascinates me. This is purely for information and for those with a curious nature.

BASIC USE OF A TENS UNIT

There's more to the TENS unit than muscle relaxation. It's all about the correct placement of the pads. Placing the pads the wrong way can have an unwelcome effect. But then again that's what people who use it are looking for.

Physics lesson update: the TENS unit sends small electrical currents from one pad to the other, creating a current that will cause a muscle to contract or relax, or do both. Muscle contraction in sensuous places can be erotic and lead to heightened orgasms.

If the woman is the giver in electrical pleasure, I advise her to try using the pads on herself to start with. That way she knows what it feels like, and she will find out how the intensity settings actually work. It will allow her to know how to make her partner feel good. The secret is in applying the right amount of electrical pressure.

Body and Soul

The electric charge is distributed across the body—not just the genitals, which is good. It means she can experience pleasure all over.

She starts by placing one pad on top her thigh muscle and one pad a little lower down, as a good indicator to how it feels on a big muscle. The stimuli react differently on larger muscles in comparison to smaller muscles. Larger muscles easily handle the current. Men have good fun trying out the TENS and making different muscle groups do funny things. It's a pleasure toy for couples too.

Once a woman has experimented with her own body, it is time to start some intimate play with her partner. She should start out slow and not forget to communicate with her partner throughout their time together. She should then slowly amp it up because there are tons of fun to TENS unit pleasure. Once she has learned the basics, she can amp up the fun.

When it comes to pleasure, there are sensuous places that are well suited for electrical stimulation. Vulvas and penises are highly sensitive and handle the pads very well. Placing a pad on either side of the vulva opening or on either side of the clitoris can induce a lot of fun. For men, placing a pad on the perineum and on the frenulum will create shockwaves of pleasure.

It might be a wise to shave those areas, mainly because the TENS pads are sticky, like on a sticky bun sticky. Applying the pads won't be a problem as they will stick; removing them, however, could cause some discomfort if the area hasn't been shaved beforehand. Ouch! Unless one enjoys that kind of pain.

She should make sure the pads are flat across the entire surface. If there are creases or folds in the skin, they should be smoothed out before applying the pads again. If the pads do not stick completely, there might be some unwanted and unexpected embarrassment.

As mentioned, she should start slowly and take it easy because TENS stimulation can be described as prickly, buzzy, massaging, throbbing, and even suckling, depending on where the dial on the TENS unit is set. This can be administered rhythmically, to music, or through a constant buzz or anything in between, and this is so much fun!

> **Body and Soul**
>
> Sex can do funny things. When aroused, her nerve endings tingle, the hair on the back of her neck stands up, and she may even get goosebumps. Her heart beats faster and her body temperature shoots up. Her nether parts feel like they are on fire! And when two bodies that are so on fire touch and move together, the heat turns into an inferno. Intimacy and sex creates lots of energy. In fact, electric sex is energy.

RISKS OF TENS MACHINES

For most people, TENS machines are safe with no side effects. If a person has allergic reactions or the skin becomes irritated, hypoallergenic pads are available in medical stores. Having said that, not everyone should play with TENS—or electrical play. A woman should seek medical advice before engaging in electro play if:

- She has a pacemaker or another type of electrical or metal implant in her body.
- She is pregnant, or there's a chance she might be pregnant, and certainly not in early pregnancy.
- She has epilepsy or a heart problem.

Never place the pads over:
- the front or sides of the neck
- the temples
- the mouth or eyes
- the chest and upper back at the same time
- irritated, infected, or broken skin
- varicose veins
- numb areas

It should go without saying not to use any electrical play in context with water, but let's say it just to be on the safe side. A small amount of water-based lube is fine though!

Tip: If a woman is in a relationship where she does not need to use a condom during sex, using the TENS unit can be fun. She places one pad on the perineum and one above the clit, and turns on the unit while engaging in sexual intercourse. It will probably blow her mind!

Special Disclaimer Note: Generally speaking, TENS units are very safe and an excellent way for beginners to experiment with electrical play. A woman can discover what she and her partner enjoy, in any way they find comfortable. I am not responsible for all the happy moments they will bring to one another with the TENS unit. But they must use it responsibly, safely, and considerately. The point is to have fun and remain safe in sexuality.

THE VIOLET WAND

The Violet Wand is the sexual version of the TENS unit. It's been on sale since the 1930s and is presently a highly interesting sexual toy. When it is held near the body, it sends out a continuous stream of tiny electrical charges and sends a spark to the recipient that is worth more than its weight in gold. I have never tried it because I'm not into electrical sex, but I thought I would mention it because other women might be interested in knowing about it.

BUTT PLUGS, PENIS RINGS, AND VAGINA SHIELDS

Other electrical stimulating toys are butt plugs, male identity rings, and vagina shields. To become better informed about electrical sex, I suggest buying *Beginner's Guide to Electro Sex Toys*. It explains the sexual electricity phenomenon.

https://www.lovehoney.com/bondage/buyers-guide/electro -sex-safety-guide

Electric-powered vibrators are as far as I go. They are the kinds that have cords to be plugged into an outlet, and are the largest and most powerful vibrators available. They tend to be a bit more expensive, but then again, a woman will never have to buy batteries.

What really makes sex great is love.

PART 6

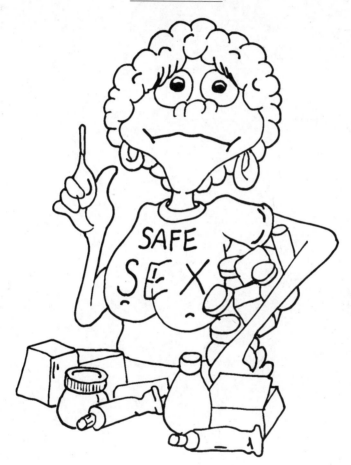

Protect Yourself

Chapter 29

Safe Sex Reminders

A woman should insist that a male partner use a latex condom for genital,
oral, and anal sex unless you are in a long-term,
mutually monogamous relationship.

What is the sexiest thing in the world to a woman? Is it when she gets up from a wonderful lovemaking session feeling good inside and outside? Knowing that she is completely satisfied and does not have a sexually transmitted disease is high on any woman's list. It is sad but true…the days of completely carefree sex have come to an end. There are cures for some sexually transmitted diseases with medical treatment; however, penicillin and other antibiotics provide no cure for genital herpes or HIV.

Part of being a great lover is taking responsibility for personal protection from serious incurable diseases. Even though total abstinence is one means of protection, it is not an enjoyable solution for the sexually active women.

> **She Should Know**
>
> BYOC: Bring Your Own Condoms. She shouldn't rely on a partner to have condoms, dams, or lube. She should always have her own supply and check the expiration date before use.

If a woman and her lover have had sex exclusively with each other for at least five to ten years, and neither has used drugs intravenously or had a contaminated blood transfusion, she can happily and safely enjoy most all the sexual treats in this book. This is often the case for the vast majority of monogamous women who read my books.

Usually, when I ask women what the sexiest thing in the world is, they do not immediately say birth control. It should be. Some of the best sex in the world is the kind that happens when couples are relaxed, confident, pleasurable, and safe. Nothing is tenser for a woman than worrying about an unwanted pregnancy and a sexually transmitted disease. Nothing is more bothersome than the worry associated with "Am I ovulating?" "Did I take my birth control pill?" "Did I bring a condom?" "Did I bring my diaphragm?" "Was that a sore on his penis?"

When she is prepared and has effective contraception, she can focus on the pleasure of her sexual experience more than the negative association that comes with forgotten birth control or unprotected sex.

Thank God, we have become scientifically and technologically advanced in both areas, and we have many options. Because birth control is safe, easy to use, and effective, couples can fully focus on the pleasure sex provides. The methods require little or no effort, and the protection is long lasting.

SHARING SENSUOUS MOMENTS

I am not going to lecture readers, but if a woman and a man are relatively new to each other, there are plenty of safe ways to share some very sensuous moments.

They should take the time to get to know one another, and then she can establish the fact that she is concerned about each participant's health and well-being. They should verbally share with one another their sexual history and intravenous drug use, and agree on what should be done to protect each other. At the very least, a woman should use condoms as a natural part of lovemaking each time she decides to have sex. It is better to be sensuously safe than seriously sorry.

EASY METHODS OF BIRTH CONTROL

Depo-Provera
What it is and how it works: Depo-Provera is a prescription injection known by most women as "the shot," containing a progestin hormone that is given every three months at a doctor's office. This injection prevents ovulation and changes a woman's cervical mucus and the lining of the uterus to help prevent pregnancy.

> ➤ **Side effects:** It has a few side effects. The most common complaint is spotting and irregular bleeding during the first year. Over time, there is no period at all while using this method, and it might possibly take several months for her cycle to return after discontinued use of the Depo-Provera. It is 99-percent effective for preventing pregnancy but does not protect against STDs.

Intrauterine Device
What it is and how it works: An intrauterine device (IUD) is a small, thin device that is placed in the uterus by a healthcare provider to prevent pregnancy. There are two types of IUDs. The **ParaGard** is

a T-shaped; copper intrauterine device that prevents the man's sperm from fertilizing the woman's egg. It provides up to ten years of protection. The **Mirena** IUD is made of plastic and works by releasing a progesterone-type hormone in continuous low doses. It provides five years of protection.

➤ **Side effects:** The IUD is 99-percent effective and is very safe. It is easily inserted and removed by a doctor. It provides long-term, trouble-free protection. It does not protect against STDs, so it is best to use a condom with it.

➤ **Specific Problems With IUD's:** Some women have side effects after getting an IUD. They usually go away in about three to six months, once their bodies get used to the guest in the uterus. If a woman can stick it out for a few months, her side effects usually ease up. Side effects might include:

- pain when the IUD is in
- cramping or backaches a few days after the IUD is put in
- spotting between periods
- irregular periods
- heavier periods and painful menstrual cramps

Pain medicine can help with cramping. If the bleeding or cramping gets pretty bad and doesn't seem to get better, the woman can inform a nurse or doctor about what's going on.

IUDs do not protect against STDs. While IUDs are one of the best ways to prevent pregnancy, they do not protect against sexually transmitted infections. Using a condom every time a woman has sex reduces the chance of getting or spreading STDs. It's best to use condoms with an IUD.

Rarely are side effects serious.

NuvaRing

What it is and how it works:
The NuvaRing is used in the same way as a diaphragm, but it remains in place for three weeks. The NuvaRing is two inches in diameter and is a one-size-fits-all, flexible, transparent ring that is placed into the vagina for three weeks. The ring is removed during the fourth week,

Watch Out

She should work toward being able to talk more candidly about sex and sexual health with friends and partners. It's easier for her to be safe when she doesn't feel ashamed.

causing the woman to have her period. While inside of the woman, it releases a steady dose of estrogen and progestin to prevent release of an egg and reduce the mobility of sperm. The ring contains the same hormone as the birth control pill. After her period, the woman inserts a new ring. NuvaRing is 99-percent effective.

➤ **Side effects:**

- ❦ Lumps in the breast
- ❦ Mental/mood changes
- ❦ Severe stomach/abdominal pain
- ❦ Unusual changes in vaginal bleeding
- ❦ Dark urine
- ❦ Yellowing eyes/skin

The NuvaRing does not protect against STDs, so it is best to use a condom with it.

Orthro Evra

What it is and how it works: The Orthro Evra is a small, thin patch that releases a continuous dose of estrogen and progestin, which are absorbed through the skin, to prevent ovulation and thicken the cervical mucus. The hormones are the same ones in the birth control pill. Patches are changed once a week for three weeks. Users do not wear a patch on the fourth week. A woman can place them on her body anywhere she feels comfortable, including the outer upper arm, butt, or stomach. The patches stay in place during physical activity and the once-a-week dosage is easy to remember. They are 99-percent effective.

> **Side effects:** Risks and side effects are the same as with the birth control pill. The patch may cause skin irritation in some women and does not protect against STIs. It is not recommended for women who weigh more than 190 pounds.

Sterilization

What it is and how it works: Sterilization is a permanent form of birth control. In women, doctors perform a surgical procedure called a tubal ligation to block the fallopian tubes and permanently prevent sperm from accessing the egg. When the tubes are tied, doctors burn, cut, tie, or block them. A new apparatus, Ensure, is a small, soft metal device that is placed in the fallopian tube by way of the vagina. The nonsurgical procedure causes a woman's body to form scar tissue around the device, thus blocking the tubes so eggs cannot pass through them.

> **Side effects:** The tubal ligation is permanent and difficult to reverse. It is not a viable option for women who want to have children in the future. It does not protect against STDs, so it is best to use a condom with it.

HORMONE-FREE BIRTH CONTROL

Barrier methods of protection are great forms of contraception that release hormones to prevent pregnancy. Using these methods is better when planned, so as not to interrupt sexual play.

Diaphragm

What it is and how it works: The diaphragm is used before sexual activity. spermicide inside the dome of the diaphragm and places the soft dome-shaped latex cup securely in her vulva so it completely covers her cervix and blocks sperm. Her doctor must fit the diaphragm to her body.

➢ **Side effects:** To prevent pregnancy, a diaphragm must remain in place for at least six hours after sex. It can remain in place for up to twenty-four hours. If she uses the diaphragm every time she has sex, it is 94-percent effective. With usage of the diaphragm, her risk of contracting gonorrhea or chlamydia is decreased.

Cervical Cap

What it is and how it works: Before sex, a woman places this small latex cup over her cervix to prevent sperm from reaching her uterus. Cervical caps come in different sizes and must be fitted by a physician or nurse practitioner.

➢ **Side effects:** For effectiveness, a cervical cap has to remain in place for eight hours after sex. It can remain in place for up to forty-eight hours, allowing sexual spontaneity while it is in place. When used consistently, the Prentif cervical cap is 91-percent effective in women who have never had children, but this drops to 74 percent for women who have given birth. The cap is not recommended for women who have poor vaginal muscle tone, cervical inflammation, a current reproductive tract infection, or any other type of vaginal bleeding. Using the cap may decrease a woman's risk of contracting gonorrhea or chlamydia.

FemCap

What it is and how it works: FemCap is a hat-shaped silicone rubber cap that is placed in the vagina before sex. It covers the cervix, preventing sperm from entering the uterus, and has a strap for easy removal.

➢ **Side effects:** It must remain in place for six hours after sex but can be worn for up to forty-eight hours. A woman can also use it during her period to allow comfortable sex play. A health care professional should fit it.

Lea's Shield

What it is and how it works: A woman places this dome-shaped disc made of silicone rubber in her vagina before sex. It operates by creating a suction that traps air between the shield and her cervix. The Lea's Shield covers her cervix and blocks sperm from entering her uterus. Like the FemCap, the shield has a strap for removal. It is one-size-fits-all, and no pre-fitting is necessary, but it requires a prescription from a physician.

She must leave the shield in place for eight hours after intercourse to prevent pregnancy. It is worn for up to forty-eight hours. The shield may reduce her risk of contracting gonorrhea or chlamydia. It is approximately 85-percent effective in preventing pregnancy. There are almost no limitations for women who want to use Lea's Shield for birth control.

- Very suitable for breastfeeding mothers.

- Suitable for women who cannot or do not want to use hormonal contraceptives.

- Easy to use, so many women choose it instead of using a diaphragm or cervical cap.

- Can be used as additional birth control method after forgetting to take the pill.

- A good birth control option.

➢ **Side Effects:** Despite all these advantages, Lea's Shield contraceptive has a few disadvantages.

- Has a high failure rate

- Has to be used with spermicides, which can affect vaginal lining in a way that makes it more susceptible to infections, including yeast infection or sexually transmitted diseases

- Does not protect against sexually transmitted diseases, including HIV

❧ Has to be used condoms during every sexual intercourse

❧ Comes with a certain risk for vaginal or bladder infections

Condom

What it is and how it works: The male condom is a sheath that covers the penis and catches the sperm, preventing it from entering a woman's uterus. For full effectiveness, condoms must be placed on the penis at the beginning of intercourse and should be used every time that a woman has sex. The Reality female condom is a soft plastic pouch that is placed inside the vagina before sex. It also prevents sperm from entering the uterus.

➢ **Side effects:** If used correctly, the Reality female condom is 95-percent effective in safeguarding against pregnancy. It also protects a woman from many sexually transmitted infections, including HIV. All male condoms—latex, polyurethane, and natural lambskin—are 98-percent effective against pregnancy. Only latex and polyurethane condoms protect against HIV infection. Condoms are the best method we have to prevent sexually transmitted infections.

OTHER METHODS OF BIRTH CONTROL

Abstinence

What it is and how it works: Depending on a woman's personal preference, abstinence can mean either saying "no" to anything sexual or avoiding vaginal intercourse. True abstinence, however, safeguards her from a potential pregnancy and sexually transmitted infections because it requires that she avoid vaginal intercourse, anal intercourse, or any other act that might put her in contact with a man's sperm.

➢ **Side effects:** Abstinence is the only method that has proven to be 100-percent effective against pregnancy and sexually transmitted infections.

Birth Control Pill

What it is and how it works: An oral contraceptive contains the hormones estrogen and progestin. The most common type, the combined synthetic pill, suppresses ovulation. The progestin-only variety, the mini-pill, alters the cervical mucus to make it difficult for the sperm to enter the uterus.

➤ **Side effects:** Some women complain of such side effects as weight gain, breast tenderness, moodiness, vaginal dryness, and a decreased sex drive. Often changing the prescription takes care of the problem. Users of the mini-pill tend to have fewer side effects. The pill is 99-percent effective in preventing pregnancy but does not prevent sexually transmitted diseases.

One of the most buzzed-about parts of the Affordable Care Act is the contraceptive mandate, which requires private health insurance plans to cover birth control without a co-pay or deductible. In other words, for free.

Chapter 30

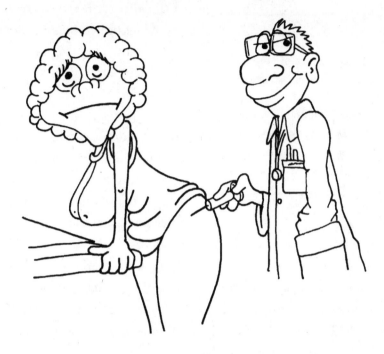

Sexually Transmitted Diseases

There are more than twenty-five diseases transmitted through sexual activity.

Sexually transmitted diseases (also called STDs or STIs for sexually transmitted infections) are infections that are transferred from one person to another through sexual contact. According to the Centers for Disease Control and Prevention, there are over fifteen million cases of sexually transmitted disease cases reported annually in the United States. More than twenty-five diseases are transmitted through sexual activity. Other than HIV, the most common STDs in the United States are chlamydia, gonorrhea, syphilis, genital herpes, human papillomavirus, hepatitis B, trichomoniasis, and bacterial vaginosis. Adolescents and young adults are the age groups at the greatest risk for acquiring an STD. Approximately nineteen million new infections occur each year, almost half of them among people ages fifteen to twenty-four.

> **Watch Out**
>
> She should choose partners who do not put all of the responsibility for safer sex on her. She should look for partners who are comfortable putting safety discussions on the table. Its safer to share the concerns.

Some STDs can have severe consequences, especially in women, if not treated, which is why it is so important to be tested for STDs. Some STDs can lead to pelvic inflammatory disease, which can cause infertility; while others may even be fatal. Refraining from sexual activity prevents STDs. Using certain types of contraceptive devices, such as condoms, can aid in preventing STDs if used properly.

Now that a woman understands more about all the sexy, exciting, and wonderful things she can do to improve her intimate relationships, she is probably ready to dive right in and have some fun. I am the first to say, "Get busy, girlfriend." Before she gets busy, though, she should stop long enough to give thought to how to really enjoy safe sex.

It is important that she learns as much as she can about sexually transmitted infections and how to prevent them. It starts before she has sex of any kind, with anyone. The good news is that, with the wide variety of fun safety gear that is available, there is no reason not to have safer, healthier, wilder, fabulous sex every time.

FYI ABOUT SEXUALLY TRANSMITTED INFECTIONS

Bacterial Vaginitis

What it is and how it works: Bacterial vaginitis (BV) is sometimes characterized by vaginal irritation and discharge. It results from a change in the different types of bacteria in the vagina. Although it's not always due to intercourse, sexually active women run a higher risk of developing this condition.

> ➤ **Does she have it?** Her gynecologist is her best friend in times such as this. He or she can determine if she has BV by performing a pelvic exam, testing her vaginal secretions, and examining a sample of her vaginal tissue under a microscope. Although many women have no symptoms, the most common are vaginal discharge and a strong, unpleasant vaginal odor.

> ➤ **How to treat it:** BV is treated with antimicrobial creams. Condoms may reduce the risk of developing BV.

Chancroid

What it is and how it works. Chancroid is a condition caused by the bacterium Haemophilus ducreyi. It is common in the United States.

> ➤ **Does she have it?** A woman might notice one or several painful ulcers on the opening of her vagina or vulva. Also, she might have swollen lymph nodes (glands) seven days after contact. Her doctor will diagnose her by performing special cultures.

> ➤ **How to treat it:** It is treated with antibiotics. Patients are examined three to seven days after treatment begins to see if it has been successful. Chancroids in uncircumcised men are usually more difficult to cure. All sexual partners who have come in contact with the affected person are treated with antibiotics, whether or not they have the symptoms.

Chlamydia

What it is and how it works: Chlamydia is caused by an organism called Chlamydia trachomatis. It is the most common sexually transmitted infection. Most women infected with chlamydia do not have symptoms. A few women have a heavy yellow discharge from the vagina.

➤ **Does she have it?** The diagnosis is made after a doctor performs a culture. A woman should ask to be tested for chlamydia, as it may not be a part of her routine exam. Chlamydia may infect her cervix, anus, throat, or urethra.

➤ **How to treat it:** Both partners have to be treated with antibiotics. Follow-up testing should occur three or four months after treatment. If untreated, chlamydia may cause pelvic infections, damage to fallopian tubes, ectopic pregnancy, and infertility. Condoms will decrease her risk of chlamydia infections.

Gonorrhea

What it is and how it works: Gonorrhea is caused by a bacterium called Neisseria gonorrhea. It is the second most common sexually transmitted infection in the United States.

➤ **Does she have it?** Most women infected by gonorrhea do not have symptoms. Those with symptoms may have a heavy yellow discharge, a burning sensation while urinating, or abnormal menstrual periods. Gonorrhea can affect the anus, throat, cervix, and urethra.

➤ **How to treat it:** The diagnosis is made once the doctor has taken a culture of any of the affected areas, and the infection is treated with antibiotics. Since chlamydia often accompanies gonorrhea, she and her partner have to be treated for both infections. If left untreated, gonorrhea may cause pelvic infections and infertility. Using condoms may decrease chances of infection.

Hepatitis

What it is and how it works: Hepatitis B infection is caused by the hepatitis B virus (HBV), which is spread through semen, blood, urine, and saliva. HBV, however, is prevented with a vaccination. The sexual transmission of the hepatitis A virus (HAV) and hepatitis C virus (HCV) is less common.

> ➤ **Does she have it?** Many people with hepatitis have no symptoms. Those with symptoms may experience headaches, fever, extreme fatigue, nausea, vomiting, lack of appetite, and tenderness in the abdomen. The condition is diagnosed through a blood test.

> ➤ **How to treat it:** There is no treatment for hepatitis infection; however, the immune system will most likely fight the infection successfully. Sexually active women should get the vaccine to protect from possible infection.

Herpes

What it is and how it works: The herpes simplex virus types 1 and 2 cause genital herpes infections. Herpes type 1 typically infects the mouth but is spread to the genitals. Herpes type 2 more typically infects the genitals. It is estimated that one in four Americans are infected with genital herpes. Most women and men affected are not aware that they are infected yet are able to transmit the virus to others.

> ➤ **Does she have it?** If she has symptoms, a woman may notice a sore, blister, or an ulcer on her vagina or vulva. The lesion could appear as a cluster of blisters or a tiny spot the size of a pinhead. The lesions may be painful or itch and can last a few days or weeks. The diagnosis is made when her doctor performs a culture or blood test looking for antibodies to the virus.

> ➤ **How to treat it:** There is no cure for herpes, and the virus remains in the body. There are several antiviral medications

that can treat herpes symptoms. If she has an outbreak, a woman should refrain from sexual activity with another person. Using condoms may decrease the spread of the virus but will not eliminate the risk completely because the lesions can exist in areas not covered by a condom.

Human Immunodeficiency Virus (HIV)

What it is and how it works: The HIV infection is caused by the human immunodeficiency virus, which attacks the immune system and eventually causes AIDS. The virus is transmitted through direct contact with blood, semen, vaginal secretions, breast milk, and, to a smaller degree, saliva. The greatest risk of transmission is with anal intercourse. But the virus can also be transmitted through vaginal sex and, to a lesser degree, oral sex. A woman's risk of contracting HIV from an infected person is increased if she has other sexually transmitted diseases.

➢ **Does she have it?** Two to four weeks after exposure to HIV, 70 percent of HIV-infected people will develop flu-like symptoms in the early phase of the infection. But many will not have any symptoms. More advanced symptoms include unexplained, rapid weight loss; diarrhea; lack of appetite; fevers; night sweats; and headaches. The diagnosis is made by blood tests used to detect the HIV antibody. It could take up to six months after exposure before a person actually tests positive.

➢ **How to treat it:** There is no cure for HIV, but there are retroviral medications that can delay the progression of AIDS, a fatal disease. Using latex or polyurethane condoms every time a woman has sex will reduce her risk of contracting the AIDS virus.

Human Papillomavirus (HPV)

What it is and how it works: Human papillomavirus infection may cause either genital warts or an abnormal Pap smear. Virtually all cases of cervical cancer are caused by HPV. There are hundreds of different types of human papillomavirus. Most HPV infections are benign and cause nothing more than genital warts. It has been estimated that more than 80 percent of sexually active women will be become infected with HPV during their life span.

➤ **Does she have it?** If she is infected with HPV, a woman may develop warts on her vulva or vagina that may or may not cause symptoms. When the virus affects her cervix, her Pap smear results may be abnormal. Most of these infections will spontaneously resolve themselves within a year. In a small number of cases, the virus will persist and cause cervical cancer or a lesion that may lead to cervical cancer over time. If she has an abnormal Pap smear, her doctor will follow her closely and may recommend further studies to evaluate her cervix. She should continue to see her doctor regularly until all signs of the infection are resolved. Condoms reduce the risks of acquiring HPV but are not 100-percent effective.

➤ **How to treat it:** Warts are treated with lasers, freezing, cutting, or several medications that she and her doctor can apply. Often her immune system will kick in and rid her body of the virus altogether.

Molluscum Contagiosum

What it is and how it works: This is a skin infection transmitted by intimate contact. A woman can catch it through sexual contact, nonsexual skin-to-skin touching, or shared towels.

➤ **Does she have it?** Symptoms include small flesh-colored, waxy, dome-shaped bumps that typically appear between two and twelve weeks after exposure. A doctor can determine if she has molluscum contagiosum by evaluating the infected tissue under a microscope.

➤ **How to treat it:** Her doctor can remove the growth by using chemicals, electrical current, or freezing. Though condoms reduce the risk of molluscum contagiosum, the virus may be in areas not covered by the condom.

Syphilis

What it is and how it works: Syphilis is caused by a tiny, spiral-shaped parasite called Treponema pallidum.

➤ **Does she have it?** The most common symptom is a painless ulcer on her genitals that appears from three weeks to three months after exposure to the infection. The ulcer typically disappears without treatment. Symptoms of advanced syphilis include rashes on the palms of the hands and soles of the feet, mild fever, weight loss, headaches, muscle pain, hair loss, fatigue, and a sore throat. Her doctor can make a diagnosis by performing blood tests.

➤ **How to treat it:** Antibiotics are used to successfully treat both partners. If caught early, syphilis is fully curable. In late stages, however, damage caused by the disease is irreversible. Using condoms may decrease risk of infection during vaginal, oral, or anal sex.

Trichomoniasis

What it is and how it works: Trichomoniasis (trich) is very common. It is caused by a parasite, Trichomoniasis vaginalis. Though considered a sexually transmitted infection, trich is transmitted by nonsexual acts as well.

➤ **Does she have it?** Trich often causes a heavy, frothy, yellow or green vaginal discharge that may be foul smelling. She may also experience severe itching or burning on her vulva and vagina, particularly when she urinates. Her doctor can diagnose her by examining her vaginal discharge under a microscope or by sending her specimen to a laboratory for

➤ **How to treat it:** Her physician can treat trich by prescribing an antibiotic, metronidazole, in a single dose or several days' worth. Her partner should also be treated. Using condoms prevents the infection.

SAFE SEX REMINDERS

To ensure safe sex, a woman must:

1. Obey and follow the sexual privilege rules. These are rules that she designs and enforces.

2. Never violate her lover by doing something he does not want.

3. When in doubt about sex, ask for permission.

4. Avoid sex acts that harm anyone.

5. Practice birth control regularly.

6. When playing games that involve restraint or pain, decide on a safety word that will let her lover know she wants to stop. This word is to be taken seriously and should never be used as a joke.

7. If she lacks trust in the person who wants to play the game, trust her gut instinct and suggest they get to know each other better before moving forward with any games.

8. Ask and discuss HIV exposure with her lover before any sexual activity takes place.

9. Always...always practice safe sex.

In the heat of the moment, it's easy for a man to forget the consequences of unsafe sex. If he takes responsibility for remembering to protect his partner every time, a woman will trust him, be grateful to him, and appreciate the pleasure during sex.

INFORMATION IS ALWAYS AVAILABLE

There is excellent information and many resource books in print that will help a woman find basic facts about sexually transmitted diseases and how to protect herself. I have listed several in the appendix of this book. I recommend that a woman read one or more of these books and educate herself.

When she is armed with facts, she can make an informed decision about her sexual activities. This powerful information will help most any sexually active female feel free to enjoy herself. Having sex with a man with whom she feels comfortable and safe will create some of the hottest moments she will experience during sexual activity.

It is especially important for women to practice safe sex because in a heterosexual relationship, women are at a higher risk than men who are exposed to the HIV virus. During intercourse the virus, if it is present in the man's semen, can enter into the bloodstream through tiny tears in the woman's vagina—tears that commonly occur during intercourse. Some women find it very difficult to insist on a man using a condom every time they have sex to protect her because men say condoms reduce pleasure during sex. These women are so involved and concerned about what men think and feel that they will risk their health and life to please the men.

Some condoms can limit the loss of sensitivity, which makes it more enjoyable to incorporate condoms into sex. If wearing a condom reduces a man's sensitivity, he can hold back from ejaculating before the woman is satisfied. When holding back, his orgasm may become stronger.

For most women, including women who want to have children, contraception is not an option; it is a basic health care necessity.s

Afterword: A Final Note

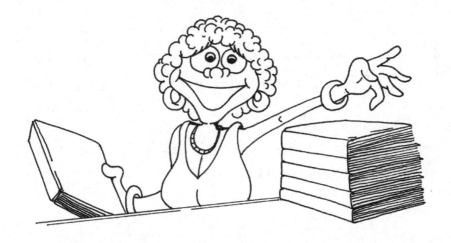

Writing this book has been the most difficult and most fulfilling, yet wildest and wackiest, adventure I have ever had.

As I conclude this book, I would like to share my own personal convictions on what I believe to be correct sexual principles. I believe that correct sexual principles are whatever feels most natural and comfortable and whatever contributes to overall good health and happiness. I understand that as a woman gets older, her views and lifestyle change and she becomes wiser in life and in love.

I wrote *Keeping the Home Fires Burning: A Woman's Guide to Giving and Receiving Pleasure* out of my sincere desire to help consenting adult women accept their sexuality in wholesome and nurturing ways.

<table>
<tr><td>

She Should Do

She shouldn't feel bad about herself if she finds talking about sex difficult to do. Many girls have been taught that talking about sex isn't romantic or what nice girls do. However, they can and they do. It gets easier with practice.

</td></tr>
</table>

This is my personal attempt to assist women in their quest for romance, sex, and pleasure. Sex and sexuality are not about performance or who has the most orgasms; it is about a woman's personal sexual healing moments. Taking the time to understand what she likes and wants from her sexual experiences will make her feel better about her sexuality. Learning what turns her on, what satisfies her, and doing wonderful things that enhance her sexual experiences are what I hope this book will do.

Every growing, maturing adult woman deserves sexual pleasure and satisfaction. She should learn about it, embrace it, and then use it to empower. Giving and receiving pleasure has many facets; there is no right way or wrong way to do it. It boils down to "what she likes." She has to take time to discover for herself what makes her feel good before, during, and after sex.

I would suggest that a woman communicate with her partner by letting him know what she enjoys, and also understand that sensual improvement is a never-ending process. So, as my knowledge deepens, more books will be published appropriately. Meanwhile, women can visit some of the websites I mention in the back of this book for the latest news, updates, and sensuous adventures.

Readers should feel free to contact me. I am open to all opinions, views, and criticisms. As always, I am delighted to hear from my readers who want to share their experiences with me. I encourage them to tell me what chapters were particularly helpful and give me feedback on how these ideas were put into action. They can offer suggestions to help others improve, as well as let me know what may still be perplexing. Although I can't guarantee total sexual success, the principles offered here are my attempt to help move women toward a more positive sexual awareness. These principles, tips, treats, and techniques have worked successfully for many who use them.

I have withheld nothing as my special secret. I have shared sensuous victories and disappointments, and as always, I wish women a lifetime of positive "keeping the home fires burning" experiences. Remember to…

- ❦ Give permission to enjoy sexual moments.
- ❦ Take charge of creating sexual experiences.
- ❦ Make rules about how to express sexuality.
- ❦ Form a sensuous relationship with the body and then enjoy the relationship.
- ❦ Celebrate sexual freedom and live in the moment.
- ❦ Free the vagina. Be sure to let it breathe each day.
- ❦ Feel good about initiating sex with lovers.

I delight in the sexual happiness and improvement of women; however, I extend this warning: be careful. By following the guidelines set forth in this book, women can outgrow the status of a beginner.

I invite and encourage women to share with me their own safe, insightful pleasure experiences. I look forward to seeing readers at my seminars. My seminars are about educating women and helping them explore their own sexuality, as well as improving their understanding. For information about conducting girl's night out, pampering parties, seminars, event pricing, or purchasing any items listed in this book, please email us at: realellapatterson@gmail.com or call us at 972-854-1824.

We waste time looking for the perfect lover,
instead of creating the perfect love.

– Tom Robbins

Appendix A: Questions for Women Who Read This Book

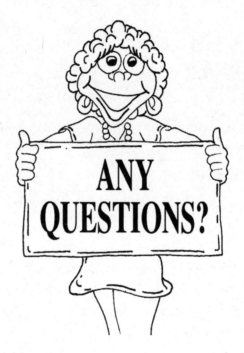

Every question does not need to be answered. She should answer only the questions that interest her. She does not even have to complete it. Just reply as she wishes to. She may choose not to answer any of the questions. She may want to create her own. Mail questions, answers, and comments to:

Attn: Keeping the Home Fires Burning
Questionnaire Dept.
P.O. Box 973
Cedar Hill, TX 75106

1. Have you had the opportunity to read *Keeping the Home Fires Burning*? Which sections, chapters, or issues do you agree with? Disagree?

2. Which part of this book is the most important to you? Least important? Most emotional?

3. Has your sensuality changed since you read this book? In what way?

4. Is orgasm easier for you since reading this book?

5. Are orgasms important to have, or do you enjoy sex just as much without orgasms?

6. When do you have orgasms? During intercourse? Masturbation? Love button stimulation? Other sexual activities? How often?

7. Do you have orgasms during intercourse? Never? Sometimes? Rarely?

8. Remembering your most favorite orgasm, give a description of how your body is stimulated to orgasm.

9. Give ways that you and your partner practice direct stimulation.

10. What kind of stimulation do you prefer? Do you prefer hard, medium, or soft massage? Do you like continuous movement? Do you like your positions varied?

11. Do you like intercourse? Physically? Psychologically? Do you have any physical discomfort?

12. Do you enjoy masturbation? Physically? Psychologically? Is it more intense with or without a partner?

13. Do you enjoy rectal contact? What kind? Do you enjoy penetration? How often do you do it?

14. What do you think about during sex?

15. Do you have fantasies? What about?

16. Do you look ugly or beautiful during orgasms?

17. Do you think that most men are uninformed about what pleases women?

18. How do you feel about your sexuality since reading this book?

19. Did you learn anything positive while reading this book?

20. Do you like objects in bed with you?

21. Do you like to use sensual toys while making love?

22. Do you have intercourse during your period?

23. Do you have oral sex during your period?

24. What are your best sex experiences?

25. How long do your sexual encounters last?

26. Do you have sex with strangers?

27. Do you usually initiate the sex or sexual advances?

28. Do you enjoy touching?

29. Who do you touch—men, women, friends, relatives, children, yourself, animals, or pets?

30. Do you feel politically inclined to have sex?

31. Do you masturbate with your partner during sex?

32. During general caressing, was it difficult to do the first time that you did it? How did you feel about it?

33. Have you discussed your sexual relationship with any other women?

34. Have you discussed masturbation with other women or not? What did they say? What did they think?

35. Do you like this questionnaire?

36. What else would you like to find out about sex?

37. Why did you answer this questionnaire?

38. Are you in love?

39. Does being in love make you happy?

40. What makes you happiest in life?

41. What is sex like with the person that you are closest to?

42. What is your biggest sexual problem?

43. What is your favorite way to spend time alone?

44. Does having children increase or decrease your sex drive?

45. How do you feel about pornography?

46. Have you ever had an affair or sex with a married man?

47. How often do you have sex with your partner?

48. Would your relationship be in danger if sex decreased?

49. How often do you want or like to have sex?

50. Does sex with your lover change for the better? The worst? Does it become boring or more pleasurable?

51. Do certain conflicts in your relationship tend to last for years or over long periods?

52. Have you found that the same problems keep cropping up even after you have talked about them or thought that they were worked out?

53. What do like most about your man? Least?

Appendix B:
Helpful Resources

Institute for Advanced Study of Human Sexuality
1523 Franklin Street
San Francisco, CA 94109

Information on Sex and Disability
It's Okay! A magazine on sexuality and disability ($23.95 a year).
Linda Crabtree, Phoenix Counsel, Inc.
1 Springbank Drive
St. Catharine's, Ontario, Canada, L2S 2K1

Erotic Aids for Women
Eve's Garden (Catalog, $3.00)
119 West 57th Street
Suite 420
New York, NY 10019
1-800-848-3837
www.evesgarden.com

Erotic Aides for Men and Women
Adam and Eve Catalog (arrives in brown paper wrapper)
One Apple Court
P.O. Box 800
Carrboro, NC 27510

Good Vibrations

(Catalog of aids, books, and videos, $1.00; arrives in plain packaging)
938 Howard Street
San Francisco, CA 94103
1-800-buy-vibe
www.goodvibes.com

Passion Parties
To find a consultant go to…
www.passionparties.com

Appendix C:
Organizations Dedicated to Sex Education

National Society for Scientific Study of Sex (SSSS)
P.O. Box 208
Mount Vernon, IA 52314

Sex Education and information Council of the US (SEICUS)
130 West 42nd Street, 25th Floor
New York, NY 10036

American Association of Sex Educators, Counselors, and Therapists (AASECT)
435 North Michigan Avenue
Suite 1717
Chicago, IL 60611

The Kinsey Institute for Research in Sex, Gender, and Reproduction
University of Indiana
Morrison Hall 313
Bloomington, IN 47405

Appendix D:
Legal and Sensuous Internet Site

- ➤ Products—www.easypleasers.com
- ➤ Products—www.stockroom.com
- ➤ Products—www.fourcuples.com
- ➤ Products—www.annsummers.com
- ➤ Vibrators—www.goodvibes.com
- ➤ Lubricants—www.passion8.com
- ➤ Sex Art—www.eroticat.com
- ➤ Sex Art—www.bettydodson.com
- ➤ E-cards—www.kinkycards.com
- ➤ Condoms—www.ripnroll.com

Appendix E:
Weights for Vaginal Exercises

➤ www.aswechange.com

➤ www.goodvibes.com or 1-800-buy-vibe

➤ www.bettydodson.com

Appendix F:
Books about Men and Relationships

What Could He Be Thinking? How a Man's Mind Really Works
By Michael Gurian

Courting a Woman's Soul: Going Deeper into Loving and Being Loved
By John H. Lee

Why Men Don't Listen and Women Can't Read Maps: How We're Different and What to Do about It
By Barbara Pease and Allan Pease

Keys to the Kingdom
By Alison A. Armstrong

Be Loved for Who You Really Are: How the Differences between Men and Women Can Be Turned into the Source of the Very Best Romance You'll Ever Know
By Judith Sherven, PhD, and James Sniechowski, PhD

Opening to Love 365 Days a Year
By Judith Sherven, PhD, and Jim Sniechowski, PhD

The Maiden King: The Reunion of Masculine and Feminine
By Robert Bly and Marion W. Woodman

Men Talk: How Men Really Feel about Women, Sex, Relationships, and Themselves
By Alvin S. Baraff

Appendix G:
Space for Private Notes

Acknowledgments

This book is a personal self-help book of the author; however, I attribute experiences gained while doing my research to many people who had the courage to tell me their stories. I am indebted to women who over the past twelve years knowingly and unknowingly contributed to this data. Numerous others helped by encouraging me to keep at it. They gave me honest and open criticisms every time I threw something new at them.

They allowed me tremendous freedom of speech, and without their faith in me I would not have been challenged to dig so deeply, probe so many crannies, or look beyond readily available answers. Without their knowledge and experiences, this book would not exist.

In many of my books, I have tried to use this page to thank people who have helped me keep it together. As I wrote this book, I recall wonderful words of wisdom received from people who empowered me. These gracious experts inspired me with their sensuous stories, wholesome levels of sensuality, and fun-loving comments. I would like to say thanks to each of them.

My gratitude goes to single and married women, lesbians, transvestites, exotic dancers, teachers, coaches, bartenders, managers, doctors, lawyers, college students, and preachers for their undying support and encouragement to this project.

To my husband, Martin Jr., thanks for being the one to say, "Keep at it, baby. You'll get it done." I appreciate you so much.

To my children, Juanna, T'Juanna, and Martin III, I continue to love each of you, and I thank you for showing me support in everything I set out to do.

To Robert Corley, this book would not be if it were not for your insight, true opinions, and support. Thanks for traveling this road with me. You are my confidant, my friend, and my truth.

Herbert Jones Jr., my oldest brother, thanks for being here—seen and unseen—to give me love, strength, and encouragement. In addition, thanks for helping me find my way. You nurtured my spirit and gave me support when I needed it most. You have never let me down, and I am so proud of you. I love you dearly.

My brother Richard Renord Jones in love and spirit, I miss you so much. I miss having someone around who looks like me. I know that God and his angels are in great company. I will be seeing you one day.

My sister Evelyn (Muff), may God be with you in all that you do. I love you dearly, even though we don't see each other much.

To my eternal friends Marva Houston and Carol Murray, the two of you have been there with me from the very beginning. I appreciate you both. Thanks for keeping it real and telling me like it is. Only true friends would do that.

My friend Betty Artis, thanks for bringing the undying support. You are a lifesaver. You stuck with me when I needed a friend most.

My friend Denella Ri'chard, thanks for your loving support and wild ideas. You gave me inside knowledge about the universe. We have laughed, stressed, cried, and planned our lives together. Thanks for being there in good and bad times.

My Soror, Brenda Brown, thanks for being an inspiring wild woman. You reminded me…that if I do not watch out, my stock will go down. Girl, you are wild and smart and always on target. I love you, Soror.

My special Soror, Debra Martin, you always keep in touch by sending an email, making a phone call, or just popping up. Thanks for reaching out to me, and thanks twice as much for showing the love. You have been so loyal to me, and I really appreciate you.

Big Boom: thanks for awakening my writer's spirit. Ghostwriting your books *If You Want Closure in Your Relationship, Start with Your Legs* and *How to Duck a Suckah* helped me get back on track. I respect your difference and forward thinking. Congrats on your book deal.

Special thanks, Larry Strader, my graphic artist. You are my behind the scenes hero.

Jan Miller-Rich, my literary agent, thanks for not pressuring me when I was going through some life-changing ordeals. Time has passed and things have changed, but your patience is my blessing in disguise. We have had times when we misunderstood one another, but that is okay because our lives have purpose, and a whole lot of other stuff we cannot explain. I really do love you for the lessons. I will never forget when we became joined at the hip. Thanks for your unwavering support. You have greatly contributed to my growth, and I thank you for it.

Allie Woodlee, my dream editor. I prayed for you, Allie. After looking over your edits, I knew God had sent me the right person. You understand my purpose, my journey, and my dream to help women. You get it, and you get me. Thank you for understanding.

Heather King, we have only worked together a short time, but I know that you are a team player and I like your team spirit. Thanks for keeping me on track. I appreciate you more than you will ever understand.

Barbara Beasley, your work is detailed, specific and needed. Thank you for proof reading my manuscript and getting in my head in the best way. Thank you for the lessons.

Austin Miller, you are family. Thank you for believing in me. I appreciate your time, efforts, and team work.

Nena Madonia, Thank you for being my hidden angel. I appreciate you.

Debra Englander, you stuck with me from beginning to end. I appreciate you. Thank you.

My God, as always, I thank you daily. I look to you for guidance, strength, and wisdom while on my journey through this life. Thanks for shining your light on me. Thanks for wrapping your arms around me. I give thanks to you for my many opportunities to make a difference in this world. "God, you are my light when the world seems dark."

If tomorrow, women woke up and decided
they really liked their bodies, just think how many industries
would go out of business.

– Gail Dines

382

About the Author

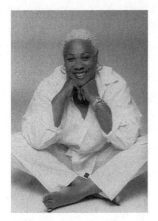

Ella Patterson is an entrepreneur, sex educator, self-published author, professional speaker extraordinaire, and columnist for several local and national magazines. She is editor-in-chief of *Global One Magazine*, and publisher of Global One Travel and Automotive in DeSoto, Texas. She is founder and CEO of Knowledge Concepts Educational Systems, a motivational company dedicated to educating and informing women to accept their sexuality in wholesome, positive, and nurturing ways. With degrees in both biology and health education, she has taught women in five countries to love themselves.

A motivational speaker for more than twenty years, she has appeared on CNN News, *Good Day New York*, *Good Morning Texas*, and every major radio station in the country. She lives outside Dallas, Texas.

Also by Ella Patterson

The Complete Guide to Sexual Healing: Over 150 Tips, Techniques, & Treats to Get Your Home Fires Burning

Will The Real Women ... Please Stand Up! Uncommon Sense About Self-Esteem, Self-Discovery, Sex, and Sensuality

Will the Real Men...Please Stand Up!: A Nine Step Plan for Lasting Romance and Passion

Moving in the Right Direction: Surefire Strategies for a Happier, Healthier and Resilient Mindset

1001 Reasons to Think Positive: Special Insights to Achieve a Better Attitude Toward Life

Ella Patterson is ready to show women how to make their relationships successful ——whether they have been married for years or are absolute newcomers. It is direct, accessible, practical, and helpful for women who want to accept and take responsibility for their sexual happiness.

A woman will learn...

...hundreds of tips, techniques, and treats that nurture her mind, body and spirit.

...secrets that help her become more sensuous, sexy, and loving.

...tips about how to get in tune with her sexual needs.

...to enhance her sexual self-esteem; and attitude for a caring and loving union.

...to accept love, give love, and believe that love is her friend.

A woman should...Read it. Believe it. Do it.

For more information on Ella Patterson products, call 972-854-1824